Beyond Self Resistance 15 Week Bodybuilding Introductory Mini Course

Beyond Self Resistance
15 Week
Introductory
Bodybuilding Mini Course

By

Birch Tree Publishing
Published by Birch Tree Publishing

Beyond Self Resistance 15 Week Bodybuilding introductory Mini Course
originally published in 2012, All rights reserved,
No part of this book may be reproduced, scanned,
or distributed in any printed or electronic form without permission.

© 2012 Copyright Birch Tree Publishing
Brought to you by the
Publishers of Birch Tree Publishing
ISBN-13: 978-0988082144

Beyond Self Resistance 15 Week Bodybuilding Mini Course was written to he[lp] you get closer to your physical potential when it comes to Real Muscle Sculpti[ng] Strengthening Exercises. The exercises and routines in this mini course is quite demanding, so consult your physician and have a physical exam taken prior t[o] start of this exercise program. Proceed with the suggested exercises and information at your own risk. The Publishers and author shall not be liable or responsible for any loss, injury, or damage allegedly arising from the information or suggestions in this mini course.

Tables of Contents

Introduction…Set Specific Goals. Set Measurable Goals and be Realistic. Set Large Goals

Chapter One…What is Self Resistance. Tension and Force. Dual Resistance. The Slim Ectomorph. Rep Speed

Chapter Two…How Much Tension. Tips To Consider

Chapter Three…Bodypart Analysis (Explanation)

Chapter Four….Ten By Ten Method 3 weeks

Chapter Five…...Double Impact Method Power Point Training 3 weeks

Chapter Six…… Compound Isolation Training 3 weeks

Chapter Seven…. Every Other Day Routine Plus Arm Specialization Fiber Overload Training
 6 weeks

Introduction

This mini course was developed to reveal the methods that you can apply to Self Resistance Exercises. It is designed to show you how to perform these exercises efficiently to get the body you want without the use of weights or apparatus. It will allow you to create chiseled rock hard muscles. It's been written by a guy who has gone through many trials and errors throughout the years. So I've created this mini-course so you can save time and learn from an expert! The primary goal of this mini course is to educate the trainee on how to perform these exercises to increase their strength, muscle size and shape!

This mini course isn't just a book with pages of exercises and no direction. It is a complete mini course featuring a Health and Strength Bodybuilding System! The unique thing about this program is that it will take you from where you are now and give you the tools to build a stronger and healthier body with proper instruction!

Although it is a mini course, you should not be left with more questions than answers. There are specific programs for you to follow, and within these pages I will reveal to you how to build your strength, improve your health and shape your muscles without the use of weights or any equipment at all. Think of it… you can build strength and shapely muscles at home or anywhere without relying on anything. Guaranteed!

This mini course and system of exercise isn't for everyone. This mini course isn't for the person that wants to be 200 pounds with 22 inch biceps. This is for the person who would like a higher level of fitness. For the person who want to be leaner with an increased metabolism. For the one who wants a chiseled muscled look with greater strength. Then, This system is for them!

At any point today you could turn on the television or open up a magazine to find the newest craze, or should I say short cut to weight loss and fitness. They promise results in days. It's just what it is ALL HYPE!

I will present honest and straight forward information on how to get leaner, fitter and stronger. It's also important to understand that it's a lifestyle. Exercise, Healthy Eating and Rest. There are no short-term quick fixes. It's about making a lifestyle change. Eating healthy is important! Dieting doesn't work because it's temporary. I'm not into that---it's a lifestyle that will last a lifetime!

My intent is to present to the world the most comprehensive self resistance course, this mini course is an introduction to that. As a Fitness Trainer, it is important that I present the right information. I've always been in a position where I am helping people achieve their fitness goals. How I present this information represents my integrity and honesty. That is something I will not allow to be compromised. Not now..Not Ever!

This course isn't a one-size fits all approach to health and fitness! This course is going to help you create a solid foundation so you can master resistance strength training exercises. The results will be for you to increase your strength and muscle tone. I will teach you the fundamentals of how to train efficiently.

However, Every person is different,but as you'll read later on in this book you must learn how to adjust your exercises, sets, reps and range of pull to fit your needs. At the end of this course, you'll learn how to individualize your training plan. This will help you to work with your genetics (what Mother Nature gave you) to become the finest pillar of strength and health you can be. This mini course was written to clear up the confusion on Self Resistance Training and make the process of getting stronger much easier! The strategies and methods are simple and you will be applying them to various phases easily!

Set Specific Goals

Getting fitter and stronger isn't easy. It takes work! Write down your goals. Put your plan into action and make a written commitment. By putting a plan of action down on paper, you will be able to compare and evaluate your progress. Goals when planted in your mind produce results!

The secret to staying motivated is to set strong goals—in writing. You need to focus on these goals day and night! Keep your mind on your plan. That's the only way you'll succeed! Over the years, I've become convinced that in order to get yourself in great shape you need to make up your mind to do it! I'm not saying day dream all day long about getting in tip-top shape. No one has the time for that. What I'm stating is that you have to channel your energy.

You also need to stay positive and take action. Add in clean eating and a exercise plan and you'll have a formula for success. Don't allow friends to sabotage your plan and slowly break down your willpower. Stay focused for you! If you tell yourself, you'll never see your abs…then you never will. If you program yourself with negativity, you will mess up your eating plans, miss workouts etc. It's called self-sabotage—don't do it!

Now, it's important to focus on what you want to achieve and not on what you should avoid! Don't focus on the negative, focus on the positive! I'll tell you some negative comments I hear everyday:

I can't lose weight regardless what I do.
How come everyone loses weight besides me?
I have the worst metabolism in the world.
I don't have great genetics for this stuff.
I'll never see any abs not now not ever!
I wish I could get rid of this stomach.
I want to, but I don't have the time.
I like my food too much.
I don't have the willpower (Want Power)!
I can't!

It's important for you to take control with positive thoughts and have control over your mental state with written goals. We all have 100% control over our thoughts. So, half of the battle is won! If you want to be successful in getting stronger, or anything else in life you need to reprogram your brain for success! It takes time it won't happen overnight, but it can be done. Stop saying I'll try and start saying I will do it!

Stay focused with thoughts like:
I like the way people are noticing my change.
Whatever it takes it doesn't matter I'll do it.
What can I eat that is healthy?
I have time to exercise and eat right.
I am committed!
I love exercising.
I can do it!
I will do it!

Set Measureable Goals and be Realistic

The best way to objectively measure your progress is to use a mirror and a measuring tape. The reason? The mirror is useful because you can definitely see the change. The same holds true with the measuring tape. Circumference measurements are a great way to stay on track. The worst is the scale. The scale will not give you the feed back you need. It only tells you how much you weigh and not how much body-fat you've got. Forget about how much you weigh and focus on the inches instead.

Set Large Goals

People always say "I CAN NEVER LOOK LIKE THAT" or I SIMPLY DON'T HAVE THE TIME" Loads of people get scared and think that they are too old to achieve their goals. They settle for what they think they can achieve not what they really WANT! The trainee needs to develop more WANT POWER than WILL POWER. For they work hand in hand. Trust me WANT POWER is more motivating!

Bio

Like most young men my quest for muscle size and strength started off with the old Liederman/Charles Atlas (Dynamic Tension Bodybuilding Programs. I started at 7 years of age with loads of bodyweight exercises, pull-ups, pushups and bodyweight squats. Years later I tried to persuade my Grandfather to purchase the Atlas Course for me, but he refused. So a school friend of mine showed me some exercises,and I did a version of the old Earl Liederman course which was in the very same spirit as the Charles Atlas course. It didn't take me very long to try just about every other isometric and isotonic course after that.

I took my mediocre physique and was transformed to a less than mediocre build, which impressed my, neighbors and friends. This was only the start! Most trainees spend their entire lives trying to devise something that works I'll give you the tools and all that is needed is for you to work it! However, like every young boy I tried weight training but loved my DT exercises and pull-ups. I stuck with weights for two months, and that was it! Years later I started competing in various bodybuilding competitions and did extremely well acquiring various titles.

I've even won Two Pro-Cards in Natural Federations. The INBF/WNBF and the IDFA.

This made me the only known self-resistance practitioner to accomplish this. I've heard many people on the internet and in person say that self resistance exercises do not work! Well if, these guys tried this form of training for 6 months, they would be singing a different tune!

Self-Resistance Exercises are Strength-Resistance-Training, so it does develop strength, chiseled muscles and can be used to increase endurance within the muscle's structure. I'm not saying that an individual that perform these exercises would be as big as an Olympian bodybuilder. No!

However, you'll have greater strength with power packed muscles Combining Methods with good science to accelerate muscle size, endurance and strength. I've realized that being patient in the exercise game, is a must. Strong muscles do not appear overnight. Be persistent and as night follows day it will happen.

I've spent most of my years trying to learn what is it about resistance strength training that increases strength and muscle development! I've tried these exercises so many different ways to maximize greater stress to the muscle fibers!
I've eliminated the guess work for you. This mini course is geared towards teaching you the efficient strength and physique-enhancing strategies. Here are the tools so be prepared to work hard!

CHAPTER 1

What is Self Resistance:

It's a unique type of training where one would use one limb to resist against another. A classic example would be to place your left hand onto the right wrist. Then pull up with your right as you resist with the left arm working your right bicep. When you reach the top of the movement, you push down with the left hand while resisting with the right working the left tricep. This form of exercise works the opposing muscle. On one arm you work the bicep and on the other arm the tricep.

Tension and Force

A trainee can increase their strength levels threefold by increasing the intensity of a muscle contraction. Once maximum contraction takes place training to failure isn't necessary. Now I'm not saying use brutal force here. That leads to connective tissue damage over time. This mini course allows the trainee to drive in multiple continuous tension gears that increases the contraction and force of every rep. Constant Tension increases muscle force and chiseled muscle growth. On a scale of 1-10 Ten being the hardest. 5-8 is best! That's an efficient form of training. Fast, Precise, Muscle Sculpting Tactics.

How To Breathe

How to breathe is the most common question that's being asked around the world. Simply Breathe, Nothing will happen.

Dual Resistance

There are movements where the trainee resist in a dual manner. This means that you need to resist in both directions of the movement keeping the resistance consistent. You may fight yourself at first but as you practice the movement it will become better with experience. It isn't easy and takes practice. Once mastered, you'll improve! There are exercises that work better in a dual manner than resisting in one direction. It's simple muscles work together as a single unit not by themselves.

Slim Ectomorph

Most people are on the slim ectomorph side, so it takes a lot for them to change their physique. So,Here's the basics for this type of build to benefit the most from this form of exercise:

1) You need to hold each exercise for a longer period of time (30 seconds or more). The reason, most trainees have an abundance of endurance oriented fibers that require more tension time to promote muscle growth.

2) You need to perform a range of 15-20 reps to reap the full benefits of the exercises.

3) Ideally, your body type need to exercise 6 to 7 days per week.
Train the 3 components within one training session. Endurance, Strength and Power. Which will give you the size building firepower and endurance component as well for increased muscle growth.

One of the methods Double Impact Reps increases stimulation, tension and occlusion (blood blockage) to get the muscles burning! It's one of the methods used to cause the muscles to contract harder which in turn promotes muscle fiber growth. What fibers are those? It isn't the get big fibers as we know the 2Bs power fibers, it's the fast twitch 2As. Perfect for the High Strung Hard-Gainer Type that have high endurance fibers that need extended tension times to promote capillaries within the muscle fibers for expansion and muscle growth.

THE 3 POSITIONS For Chiseled Muscle and Strength Gains

Here's a plan to increase the angle of pull that will trigger maximum muscle building stimulation.

1) Basic Exercises ....Muscle Teamwork to trigger intense contractions

2) Stretch Exercises …….. Semi Isolation exercises to increase and produce a stretch to lengthen the fibers to contract harder.

3) Contracted Exercises (Blood Blockage) Exercises to increase endurance component expansion within the muscle. (increasing capillary bedding) within the fibers to promote additional chiseled muscle fibers.

All of these components are important for increasing strength, muscle shape and muscle blood blockage to increase muscle building hormones. Pre-Stretching the muscle at the point of stretch increases the hypertrophic muscle sculpting response. So for maximum strength and size increases, stress methods should commence within those positions to ramp anabolic hormone release for the best gains.

Here are some of the exercises:

Basic……Decline pushups, three-chair dips, regular squats these trigger the greatest testosterone release.

Stretch ………Across-the-body lateral raises, across-the-body pulls. Stretch type exercise produce anabolic hormone within the muscle structures.

Contracted Exercises……Forward raises, tricep press-down. Block blood flow for muscle burn which increases and stimulates hormone release to promote and coax additional muscle growth.

Sample Plan
An Example of this protocol would be:

Decline Extensions (Muscle Teamwork works lateral head),

Overhead Tricep Presses for stretch overload (which work the long and medial head)

Reverse press-down for occlusion (medial and long head)

This is an efficient plan but if you add double impact reps (to be discussed later) your results will skyrocket! This combination is a full range muscle sculpting program. Once the muscles gets use to this it's time for a change of pace to trigger ongoing progress. That's why each plan is designed for 3 weeks only before full adaptation takes place. Which is excellent for coaxing the muscle into size and strength gains every so often. You build every facet of the muscle and trigger greater strength faster. A three to four week plan will increase vascularity and muscle fiber detail for that hard chiseled look.

Each workout will give you full blown pumps to increase muscle building growth. It's been said throughout many circles that muscles need 48 hours to recover. In truth, muscles tend to regress after a few days of non-training. Muscles don't need that much recovery time to progress. It's a classic example of one step forward eight steps back! A muscle can be worked again after 30-45 minutes of high intensity training. With this program, you're blasting each muscle through it's full range of motion. Plus you're using more volume (sets) in less time due to basic exercises(muscle teamwork) and muscle coaxing stress methods. There are split routines that work the muscles directly and then later indirectly with another workout. This speeds up the growth process.

Rep Speed

Now for the components of ideal rep speed for maximum gains in strength and muscle size. Ten- seconds up and ten seconds down or slower speeds will not produce the best in muscle building and strength gains. It's the power cadence of 3 seconds up 3 seconds down, that promotes the muscle size and strength. Forget super-slow. You'll get more fatigue producing components due to too much lactic acid accumulation and no muscle growth. It's a useless training protocol!

Later you'll see suggested routines and rep ranges for each body-part. They are only suggestions though because after the full course you'll figure out what type of tension and rep range works best for you. If not, keep going and you'll get there soon enough. Also, a day of rest between body-parts splits works very well on recovery but isn't necessary. You can train a muscle every day if you like.

Here's an example...You can combine workouts like this:

Combine a basic with a stretch movement for one workout and then for the next combine the basic with a contracted exercise for the next. This keeps the workouts fresh. That's just one example. Another strategy is to use different positions each training day. For example you can perform a basic shoulder exercise like resisted shoulder presses and resisted forward raises. The next workout would be the same resisted press but with a resisted upright row.

Change is necessary for progress to occur. The muscle-building split routines will cover all angles of pull and push giving you complete development. The methods are potent and really intense so do not overdo them! This mini course isn't a book made up of 500 mindless bodyweight squats or hundreds of pushups that will cause tendonitis and sore inflamed connective tissues, in the long run. It's main focus is creating strength, muscle balance and a beautifully sculpted physique! Strength and Physique development will only be built on medium to high resistance that impose high levels of tension and stress on the muscles.
The various phases will show you how to select exercises and methods that will be challenging. That will coax the muscles to squeeze a few extra reps.

If regular full range curls are easy then switch to Double Impact Reps!
By alternating leverage and weight distribution you stimulate great stimuli and coax the muscles to work harder! Strength and physique are developed by stressing the muscles by making the exercises harder not exhausting them with silly countless reps.

Resistance Exercises is one element of the equation the other is learning how to contract the muscles powerfully! It's better for the trainee to develop a practice mindset as opposed to a workout mindset. This is a learning phase. Mindlessly adding reps of endless pushups, pull-ups and abdominal exercises are to a point good for general cardiovascular fitness and endurance but will do nothing for building Real Defined Muscle and Strength!

Remember, Muscular Tension builds real strength not countless high rep training. Performing countless reps generates less tension and force on the targeted muscles. Strength is about tension of the contraction.

I've spent my entire life studying bodybuilding, fitness and nutrition. Ever since I can remember, I wanted to know everything there was on getting more muscular, stronger and fitter. It consumed most of my life. I remember studying all my training manuals and reading stacks of journals about physiology and nutrition. Studying every word diligently!

I TURNED MYSELF INTO A HUMAN GUINEA PIG!

I have learned that book knowledge is one thing, but true execution and experience is the only true teacher,and that was my quest. Once a trainee practices frequently they will become successful. As stated,There's nothing wrong with performing a resistance move everyday. Regardless of what conventional bodybuilding gurus say. A muscle can be worked everyday, twice a day even three times a day if one desires. However, the intensity must be moderate if one trains 2-3 times daily.

CHAPTER 2

A lot of trainees that I've shown this method to apply great tension on the first go by fighting the contraction instead of learning how to contract the muscles efficiently to promote strength and tissue growth. Antagonist/Agonist (opposing muscle training) is pretty simple to perform but hard to master! With resisted curls the biceps fight the triceps to contract and extend. Learning how to perform and master the movements won't come overnight and takes practice.
Make it a learning phase.

HOW MUCH TENSION

Tension or Progressive Resistance is the name of the game here. One needs to be careful and not overdo the tension. In order to understand we need to start at the top. The key principle the SAID principal. (SAID stands for Specific Adaptation to Imposed Demands). In short a trainee need to train with a variety of methods for the greatest amount of stimuli.

Getting a muscle to generate the strongest muscle building signal can be very difficult! With progressive resistance training maximum force is not necessary. It just needs to be strong enough. Also, Maximum tension isn't necessary to produce results with this form of exercise and is not advisable!

As before, Resistance should be between 50-70 percent to increase muscle growth. Using a scale of 1 to 10. Ten being the hardest. Resistance should fall between 5-8. Most trainees would benefit from continuous reps of 15-20 within a 6-8 set count. In most cases with this amount of tension and reps, the muscle will appear to have increases in size and vascularity.

Using resistance of 60% for as many reps as 15-25 reps are best in certain phases. To really get anywhere and prevent burnout maximum or near maximum resistance is out! Such training practices are overly taxing to both the nervous system and connective tissues. As stated before,I do agree that one should increase the overload but increasing the tension is only one element that isn't necessary to increase one's size and strength. There are other factors and components to consider as well!

TIPS TO CONSIDER

1) Stick to 6-9 sets of 15-20 reps per set most times.

2) By week two, increase your tension (resistance) slowly. It is best to learn and observe how you feel and remember if you don't feel it no real results will be achieved.

3) All or None Law--This really means that if the intensity is too great then no true contraction will take place equaling no progress.

4) Some trainees may realize especially hardgainers they need to increase the tension spent on the muscle to trigger growth so a 15-20 rep range is an excellent gauge! These trainees have an abundance of endurance-oriented fibers and need ample stress to coax muscle growth and strength. Hard Gainers are delt with poor nerve to muscle firing pathways and one of the biggest mistakes trainees make is using too much force (tension) that doesn't last long enough to trigger a muscular adaptation. (muscle stimuli) tension time on the trained muscle needs to be at least 30 plus seconds to increase muscle growth with self resistance exercises.

Your first week of working out should be easy! Not so easy but easy enough that you will get mild soreness. Break-in slowly. That will help you learn the exercises. Get in touch with your muscles and body and rhythm for training. Don't be over jealous and use too much tension within the phase as it's a learning phase. Take it easy and you will set the stage for increased gains and self mastery for the future!

These plans are set up as a Six-Day-A-Week Approach. Performing the same exercises for 3 weeks. That's the ideal frequency to learn the movements and develop nerve to muscle path ways for more complete target muscle building stimulation. Every single time you train within the first few weeks your muscles will fire more efficiently. That increase will translate into rapid strength increases.

Due to the adaptation you will realize that by the third week you will feel stronger and will be performing more reps than before! Within the third week the training will be changing and you will move to a slightly more elaborate routine that will force the body to emphasize neuromuscular efficiency. This will increase your strength levels.

The first two weeks you need to focus on learning how to contract your muscles and learn the exercises and stress methods. Always stay in control of the exercises. Do not bounce or do fast reps this causes pressure to be placed on the connective tissues as opposed to the muscles. The key is to place as much stress on the muscles as possible. If in doubt go slower! Always use a steady controlled speed not a fast one.

Use a resistance that is moderate so no strain is involved. Follow the program to the letter for the first week and the second week use a stronger resistance with no straining! Become a feel master and you will be successful at completing your workouts.

Neck Exercises

The neck muscles and upper trap muscles are the most important muscles in the body apart from the lower back. The neck is very important and supports the weight of your head that's 8-10 pounds. All the neck exercises increases the strength, size and shape to the neck. As we say in the fitness world, alinement starts at the top! A well rounded neck/upper traps routine will enhance one's posture and maintain balance for the head.

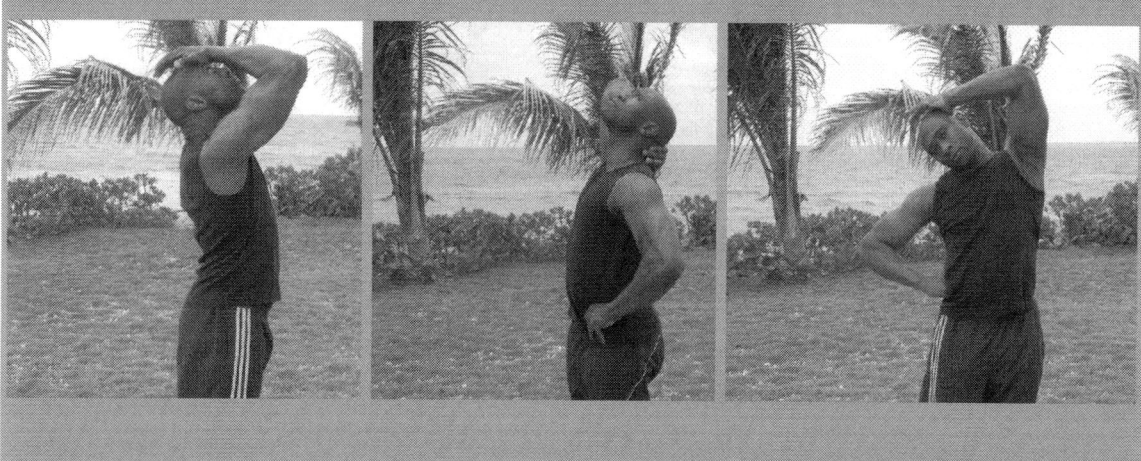

CHAPTER 3

NECK AND UPPER TRAPEZIUS EXERCISES

Front Neck Press (Stretch and Contracted)

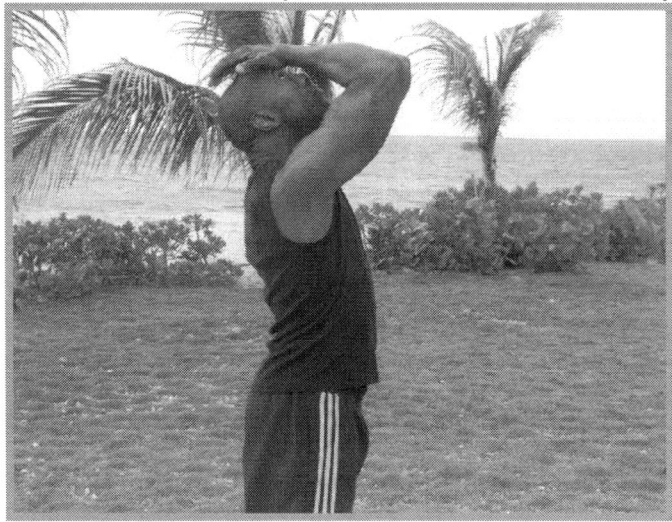

Start Position

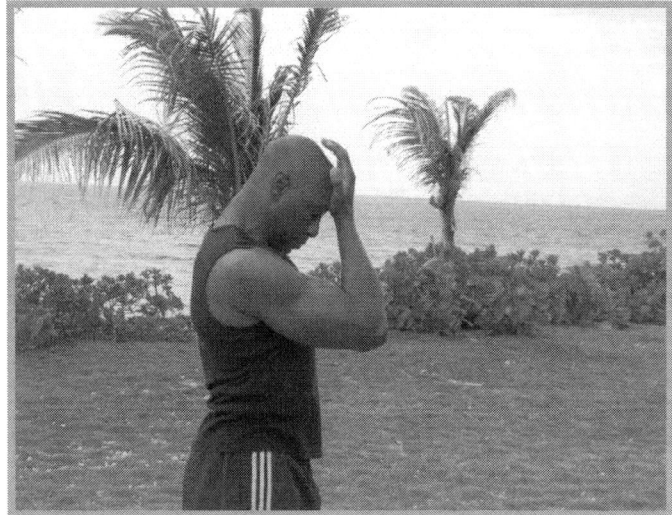

Finished Position

With your head tilted back place your hand on your forehead. Now slowly press your head forward and resist the movement slightly with light tension towards your upper chest. Always use a light tension to the neck. As your strength increases use a little more force but not too much tension. Breathe Normal.

Rear Neck Press (Contraction)

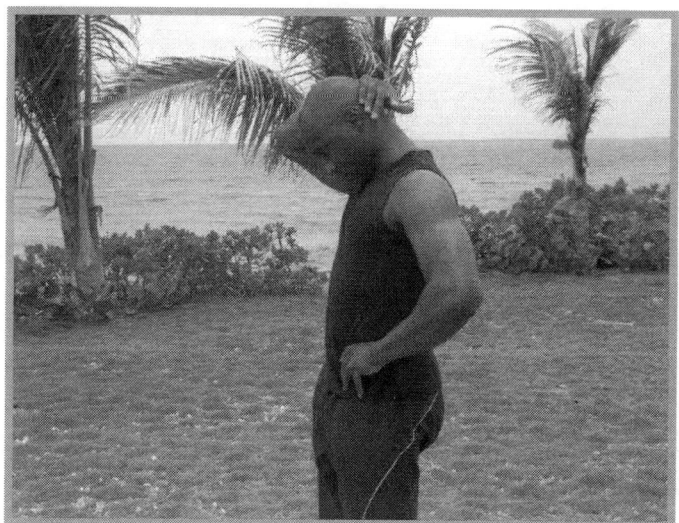

Start Position

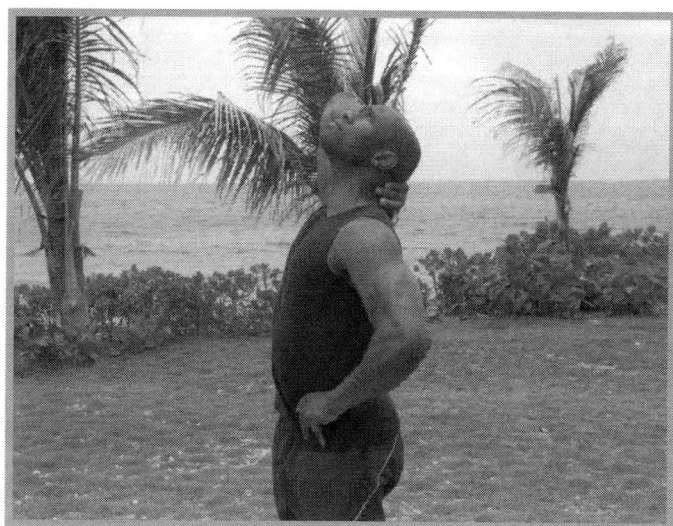

Finished Position

This movement is the opposite of the first movement. Place one hand behind your head and tuck the chin on the upper chest as shown. Now press the head against the hand while resisting with the hand until you're looking straight up. Use a light tension at the beginning and increase the tension to medium as you get stronger and more conditioned.

Side to Side Neck Upper-Trap Press (stretch)

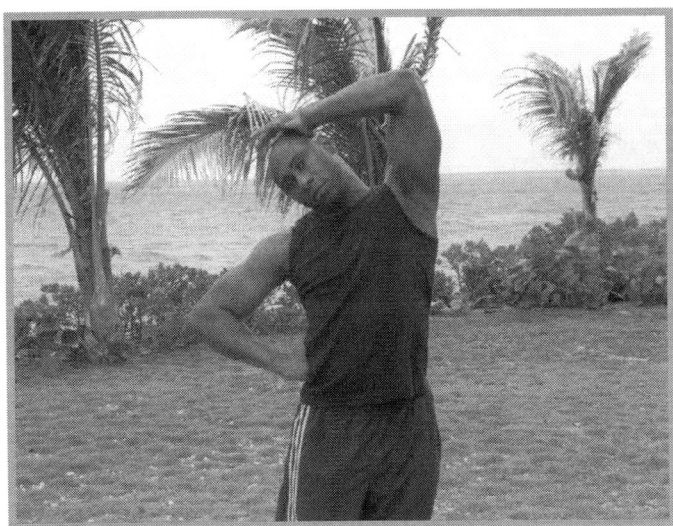

Start Position

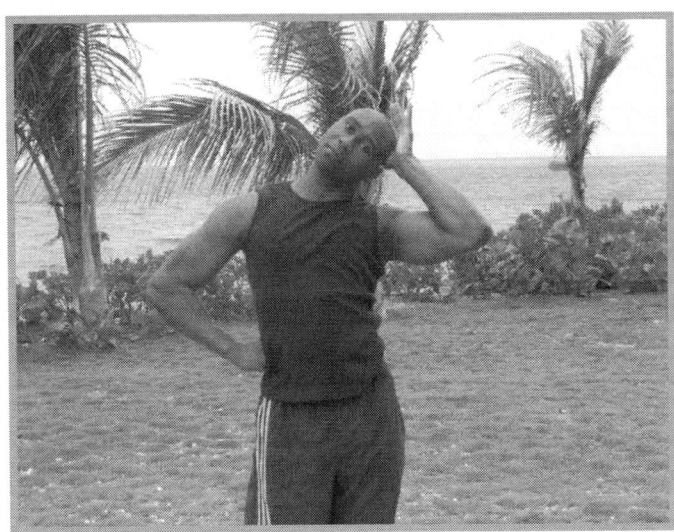

Finished Position

Bend your head as close as you can to the shoulder as shown. Place the left hand on the left side of the head and press the head to the opposite shoulder while resisting with the hand. Followed by placing the right hand on the right side and press the head back to the starting position as before. Dual action left then right. Remember use a light tension and once the neck becomes more conditioned and stronger increase the tension.

Chest Exercises

It's important to hit the chest muscles from many angles as possible to coax and force development. However, I learned that in order to really build a good chest it isn't one or two exercises it's a variety that will build the chest and increase it's strength! So in truth the best thing to do is to divide the chest in sections. Upper Chest, Inner Chest, Lower Chest. Instead of looking at it as a whole because it isn't. You must treat the upper and lower chest as two separate entities for your chest building venture to be a success. In my early years I did loads of pushups for the chest which hits mostly the lower and outer portions of the chest and do next to nothing for the upper chest. So I switched to decline pushups hands on blocks elbows in instead of out and the upper chest was taxed a great deal! So now my chest building starts with upper chest training. Giving priority to developing and stressing the upper chest.

Basic& Stretch: Decline pushups elbows in hands on a block works the upper chest really well. Along with help from the front portions of the shoulders and the tricep muscles.

Stretch& Contracted: Liederman Presses and Across the body presses really hit both elements in pre-stretching and increasing the peak contraction at the end of the movement. This position involves muscle-teamwork as well which will help the chest perform the movement. Help from the shoulders and triceps. Let's take a look at some muscle sculpting exercises.

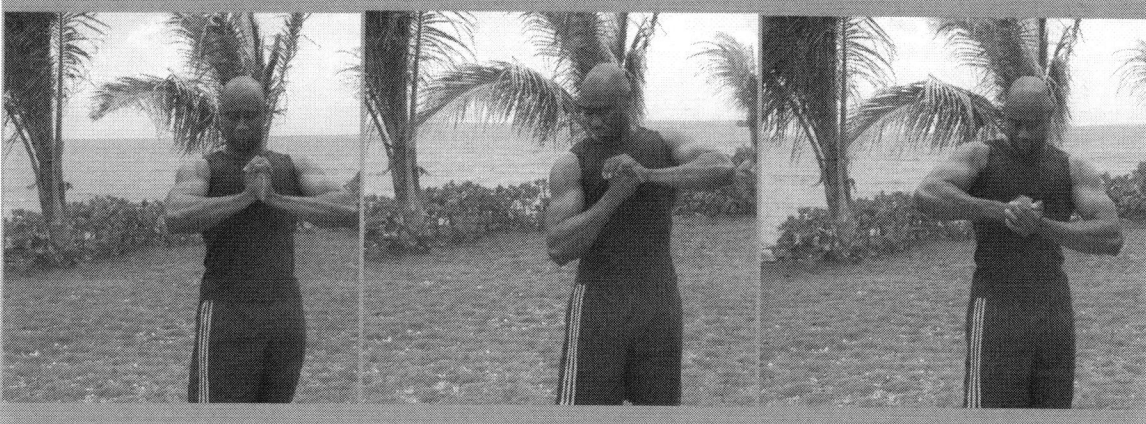

Chest Exercises

Upper Chest Press (Stretch and Contracted)

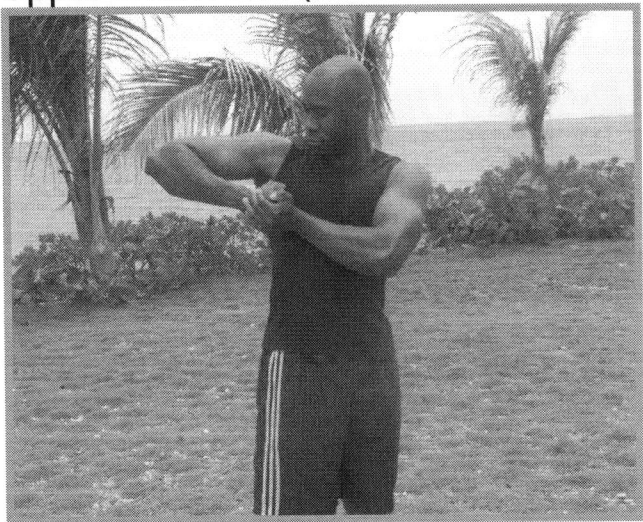

Start Position

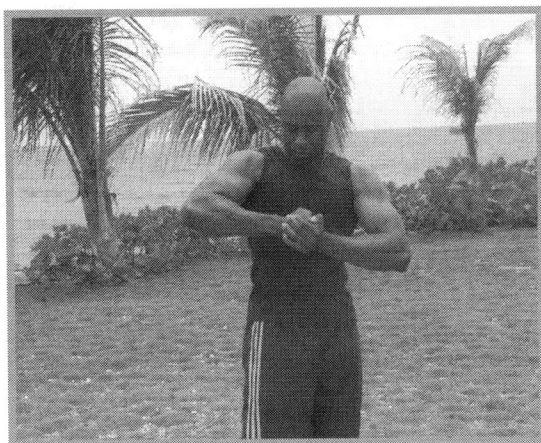

Mid-Point

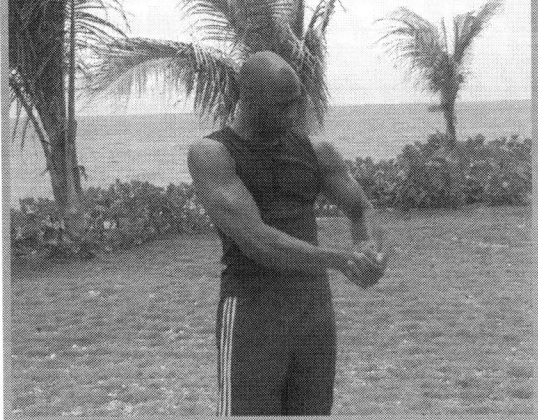

Finished Position

Place the right fist in the palm of the left hand as shown. Press the right hand down-wards resisting with the left hand until the right arm is across the body towards the left hip. Press the left hand upwards to the start position and repeat. Then change sides after all the reps are done. This exercise is a pre-stretch and contracted move.

Liederman Press (Stretch and Contracted)

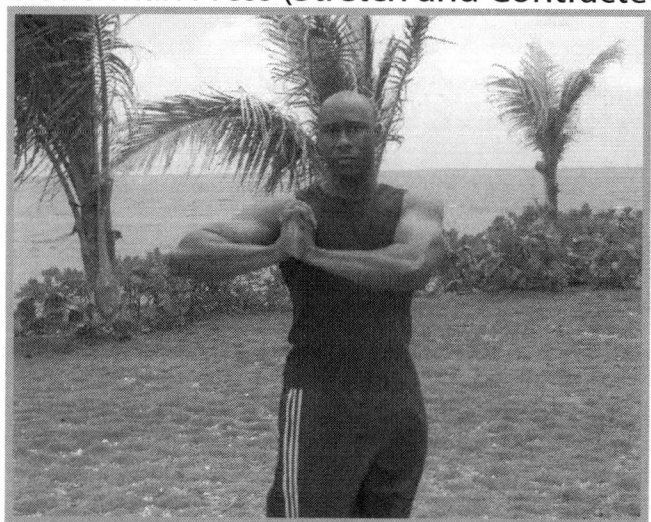

Start Position

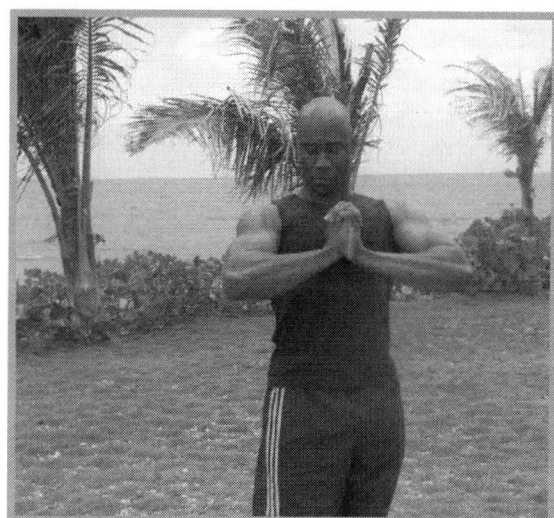

Mid-Point

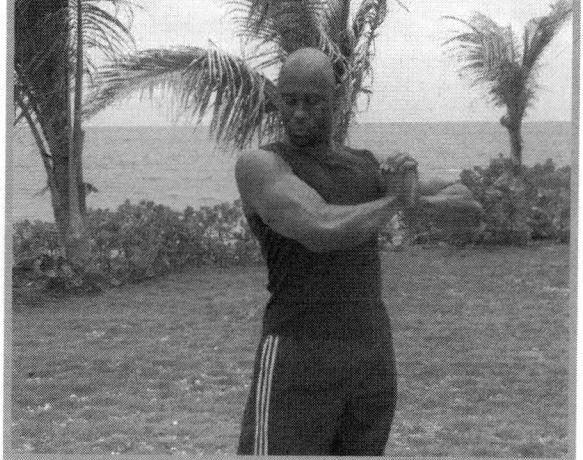

Finished Position

This is an Awesome building and shaping movement. Works the entire chest, lower, upper and middle chest as well as the shoulders and tricep musculature. Start off with the fingers interlocked as shown at the right armpit. Press right palm against the left palm towards the left armpit. Pause for 1-2 seconds and press the arm back and pause again before repeating.

Decline Push-Ups (Basic and Stretch)

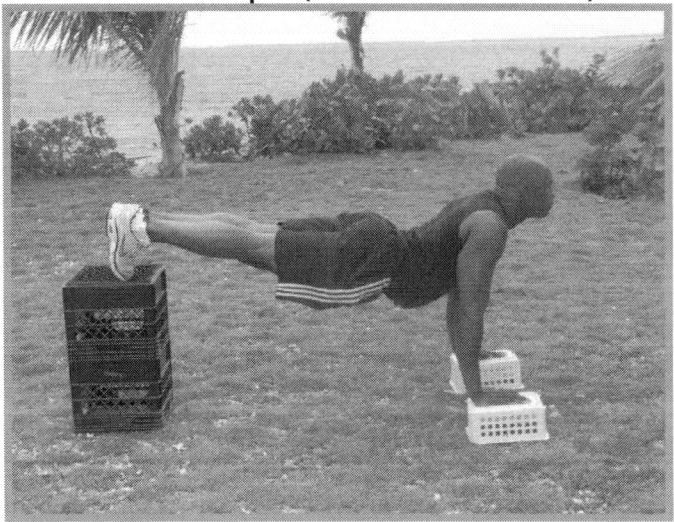

Start Position

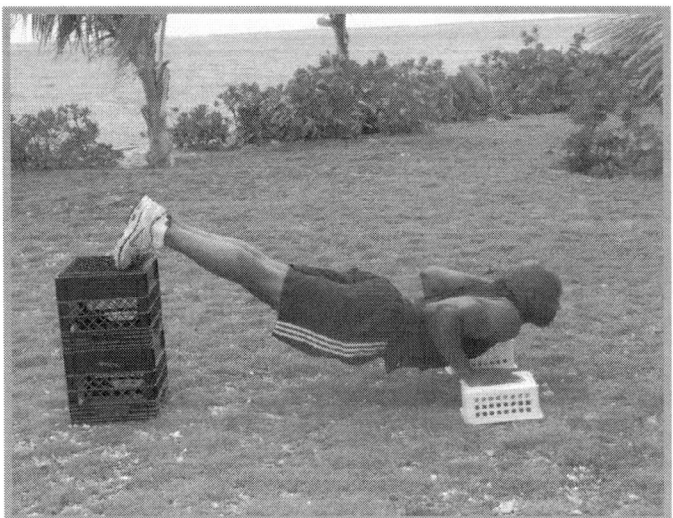

Finished Position

This exercise is the Granddaddy of all upper-body exercises. An advanced version of the original Liederman pushup. This was his key upperbody exercise for the chest. It's the best upper-body builder and conditioner there is. This exercise is performed exactly as shown. Place your feet on a chair or box that's 10-15 inches high the higher you go the greater pre-stretch there is. At the bottom position to enhance muscle building stimuli pause at the bottom for 2-3 seconds before reversing the movement. Excellent for the upper and lower chest.

Three-Chair Pushups (Basic and Stretch)

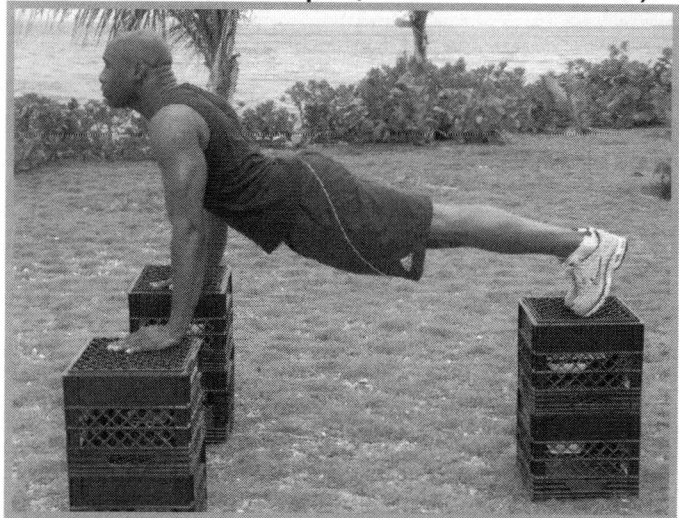

Start Position

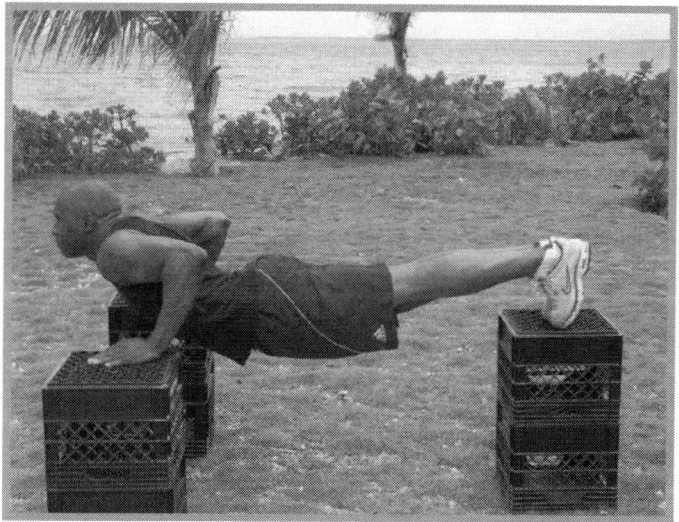

Finished Position

With three chairs as shown in the picture above, place your hands at least 15-20 inches apart depending on the width of your shoulders. If unclear, I suggest shoulder width no wider. Lower yourself to the finished position and at the point of stretch. Reverse the movement. Do not drop or dip too low.

Upperback Exercises

The structures of the upper back is quite powerful every point needs to be very carefully targeted. Basic Synergy Muscle Team Work, works well here. Thigh Rows, Resisted Pull-downs or Three Chair Dips are major corner-stone exercises to target the powerful upper back muscles. This will be explained within this chapter

Back Analysis

The upper back is very complex and house loads of different muscles coming together to form the master piece of a powerful rugged muscular upper and lower back. Now to target the bulk of the mass to the back one needs to exercise the larger areas of the back the lats, upper neck and mid back muscles. This will hit the smaller muscles as well.

The best way to start is to break things down into sections to see where what is targeting to really realize what you're doing and how to effectively target that large mass of muscle more efficiently.

Latissimus Dorsi The sides of the upper back.

Basic: Thigh Rows, these are perfect for targeting the upper and lower lat muscles as well as the lower back. Apart from that there's Resisted Pull-downs that targets the lats fully from top to bottom. These exercises are under continuous tension within the range of pull. However with the Thigh Rows resistance drops off a bit at the top position but by all means a highly effective exercise.

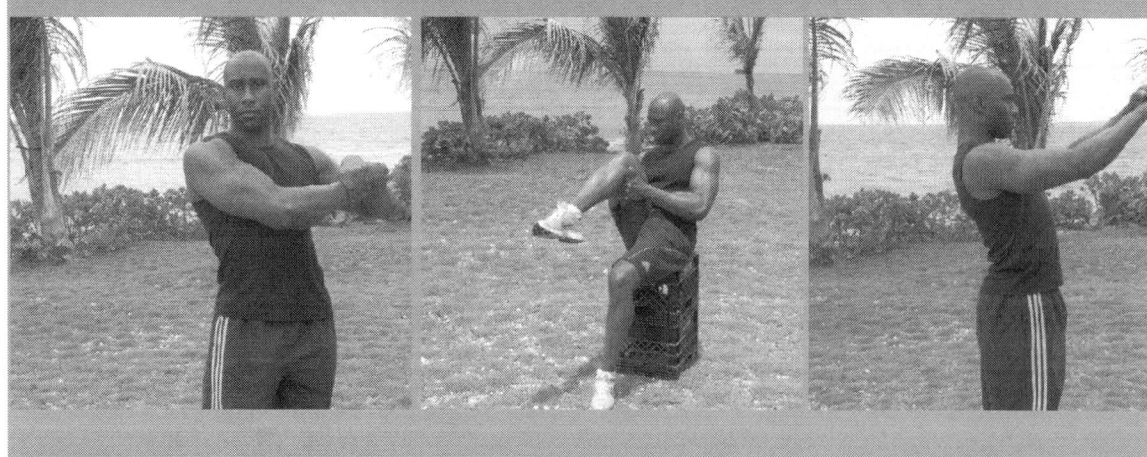

Upper/Lower Back Exercises (Basic)

Thigh Rows

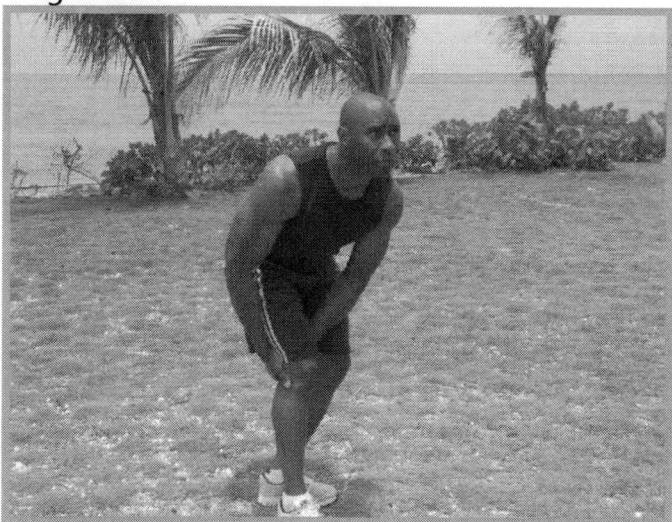

Start Position

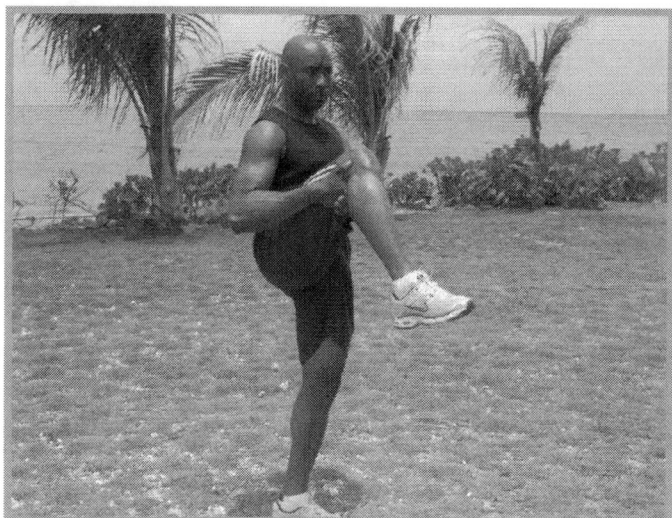

Finished Position

Interlock the fingers behind the knee as shown with right leg. With both arms pull the thigh upwards towards the chest while resisting with the leg. This exercise widens the upper back, works the mid-back and stimulates the biceps as well. Work one side fully then switch to the other side. If balance is an issue perform the exercise standing against a wall.

Three Chair Dips (Basic/Stretch/Contracted)

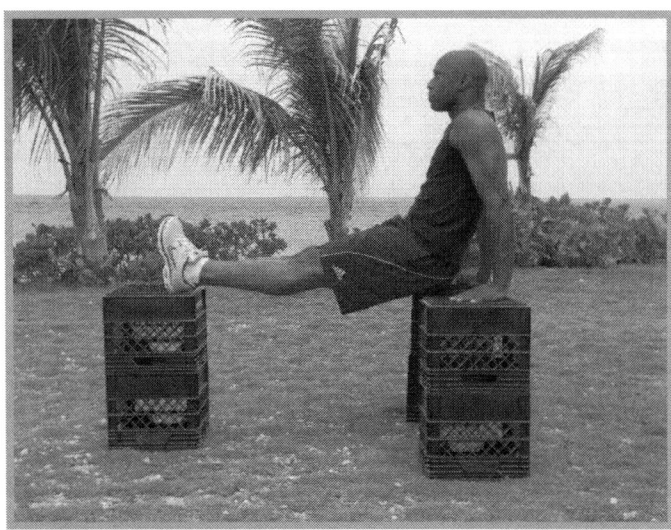

Start Position

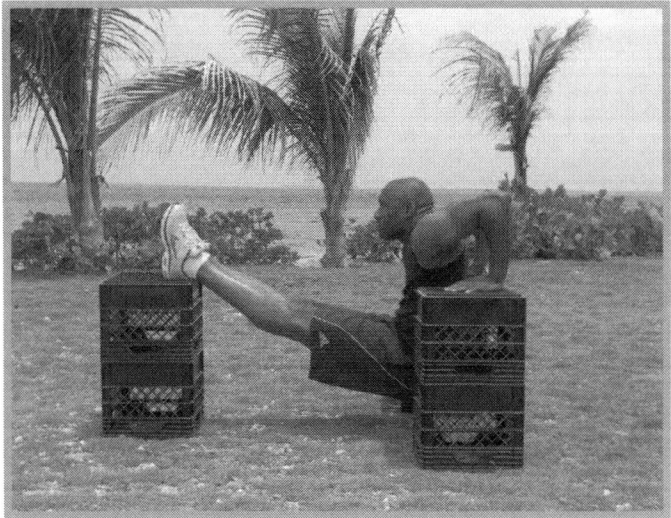

Finished Position

As shown place each hand at least 15-16 inches apart, or shoulder width. Lower the body between the chairs pause one second and reverse the movement to the starting position. This is an awesome upper back widener.

Stiff Arm Pulldown (Contracted)

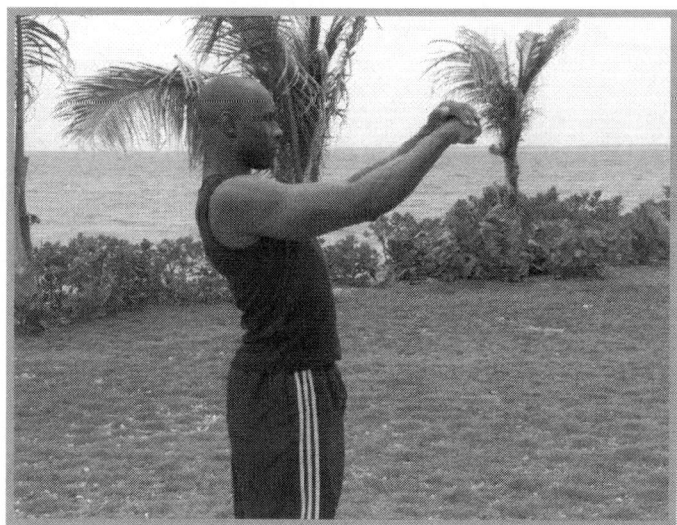

Start Position

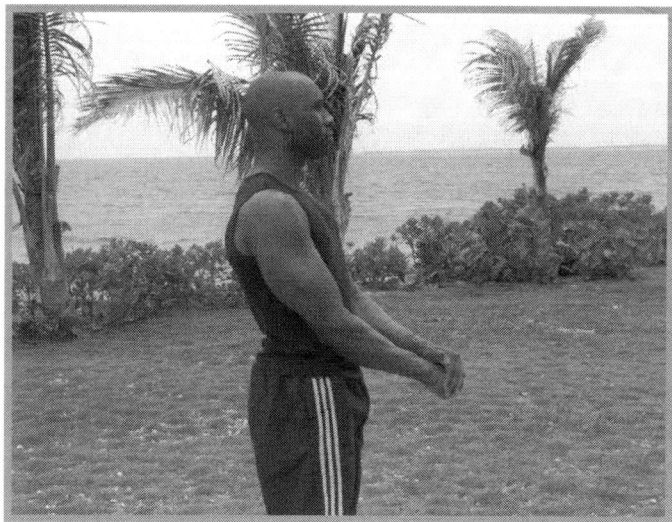

Finished Position

Grasp the left hand with the right as in the picture. Gradually pull the arm downwards while resisting with the bottom arm. At finished position, Repeat by pressing the bottom arm up again by resisting against the top hand. Resisting in both directions for reps, then switch. Fantastic Upper and mid back strengthener.

Upper-Back/Mid-Back/Rear Delts (Pre-Stretch and Contracted)

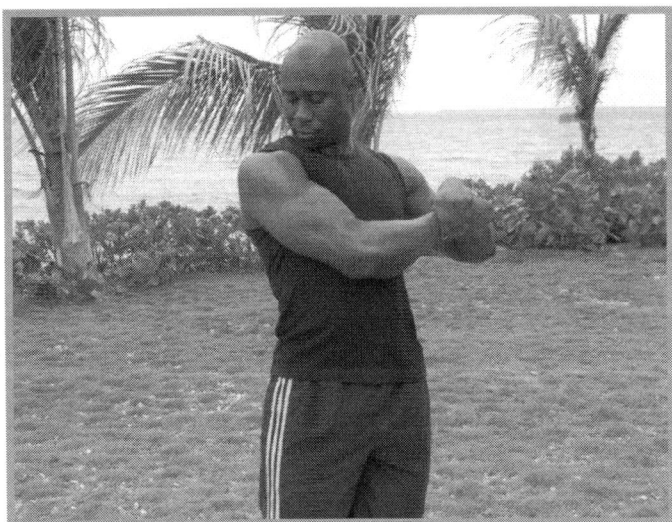
Start Position

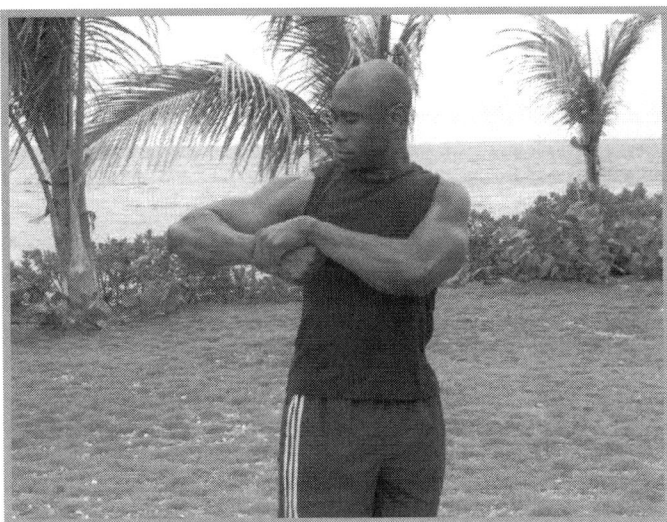
Finished Position

Bring your right arm across the body pre-stretching the mid-back, grasp the wrist with the left hand. Slowly pull the arm across the body toward the right armpit against the resistance supplied by the left hand. Repeat the movement then switch arms. This adds thickens to the mid back and lats, along with the rear part of the shoulders.

Resisted Pulldowns (Basic and Contracted)

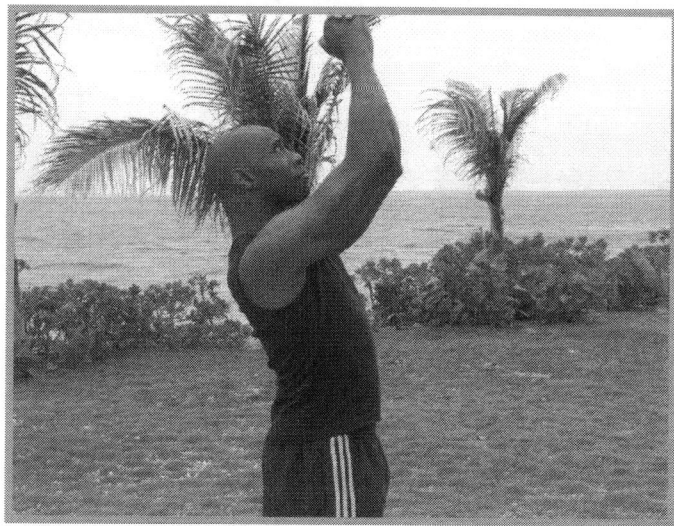
Start Position

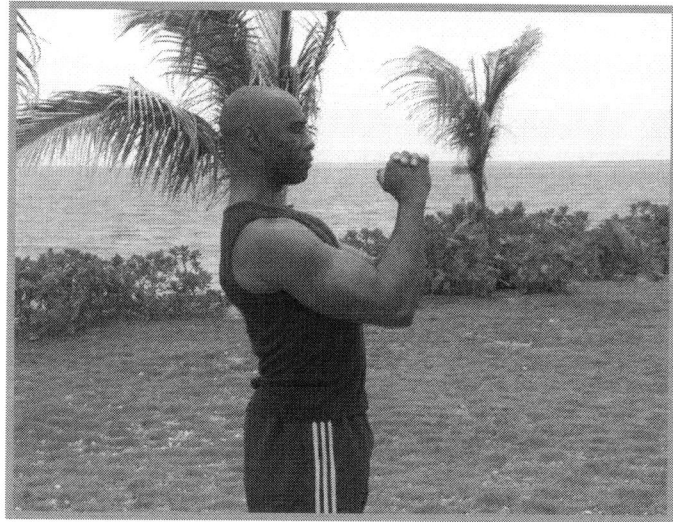
Finished Position

With the arms overhead place your left hand on top of the right fist as shown. Pull down with the left hand resisting with the right, once at finished position press the right hand up resisting with the left hand for the desired reps. Then switch arms. This works the entire upper back, biceps, and shoulders

Mid-Back Upper Traps (Contracted)

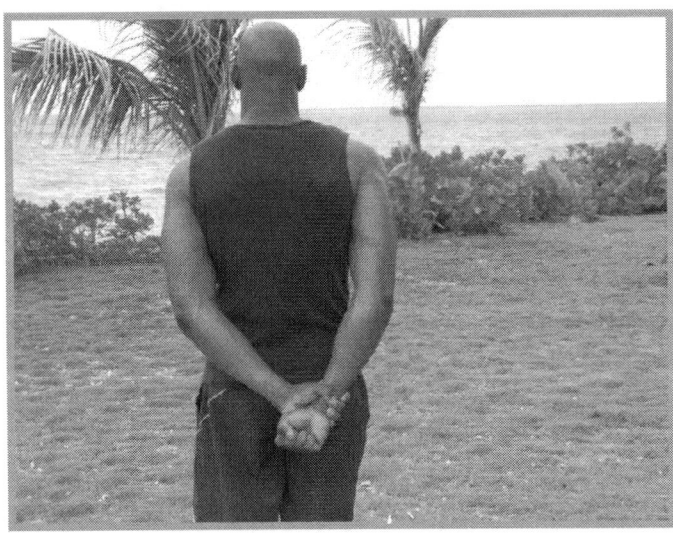

Start Position

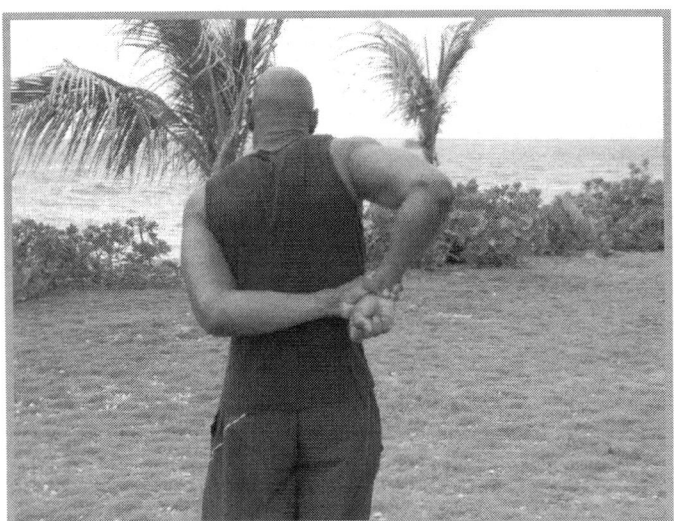

Finished Position

Place your right arm behind your back, hold onto the wrist with the left hand lean forward a-little and pull the right arm upwards while resisting with the left. When fatigue switch arms and continue. This works the mid-back, upper traps and rear delts.

Shoulder Exercises

There's exercises that directly target the side head of the shoulders giving you that wide look. However at the very start I did an exercise that was just magic in terms of side and overall muscle development and strength. It's decline pushups hands on floor (elbows out). One can perform this by itself or with the isolation self-resistance type exercises to add even more strength and muscle growth. Now it's been said that the lateral (side) will only be activated with lateral movements..but both forward and side resisted raises will stimulate the two heads.

The reason? One works with the other and they are intertwined with each other. The shoulder routine are packed with strength building and muscle pumping exercises that will create more width and roundness with efficient and muscle stimulating exercises. The shoulders contain three separate muscle heads, Front, Side and Rear heads. Lets take a closer look.

Shoulder Training & It's Effects

Now with all the pushing movements You'll be doing within this course you may think that you should lay off shoulder exercises a little seeing that almost all the upper body exercises contain some form of shoulder involvement. The shoulders, just like the calves and forearms. Constantly working. Flexing and relaxing all day long when we walk, write/type, drive, lift a bag or put something on a shelf. Just like the upper back you need to separate the sum of parts and hit them in sections to really optimize your training when it comes to that area.
Once separated precise and efficient training will surface.

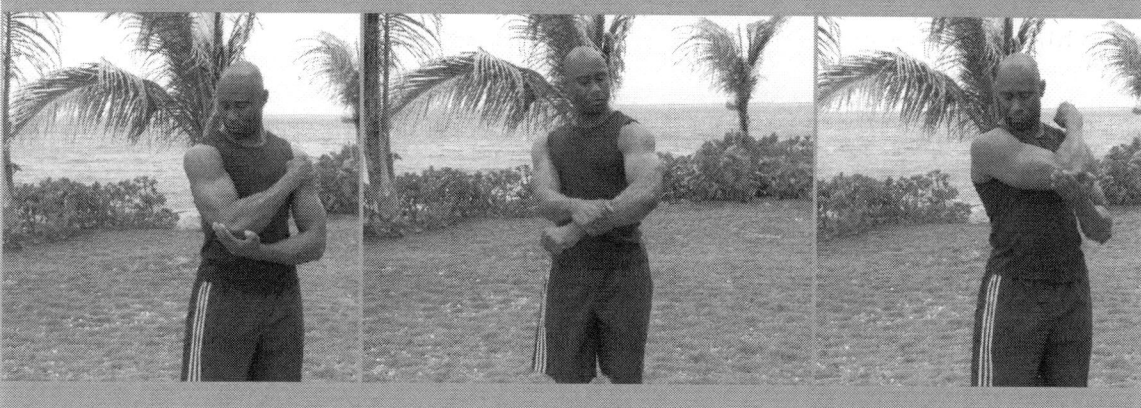

Decline Pushups (Basic)

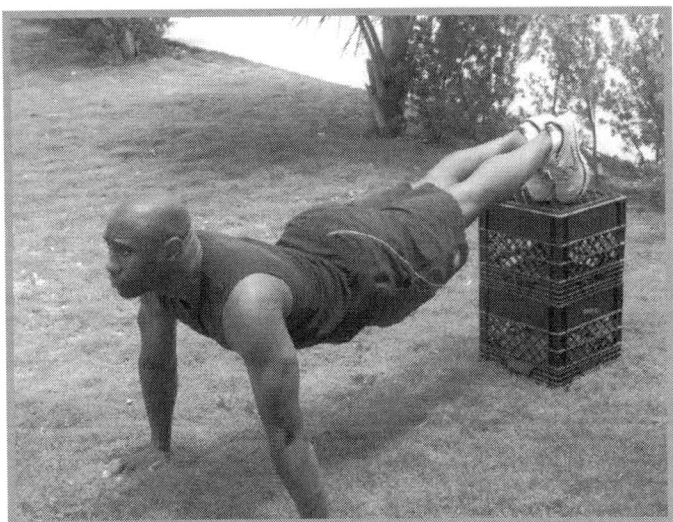

Start Position

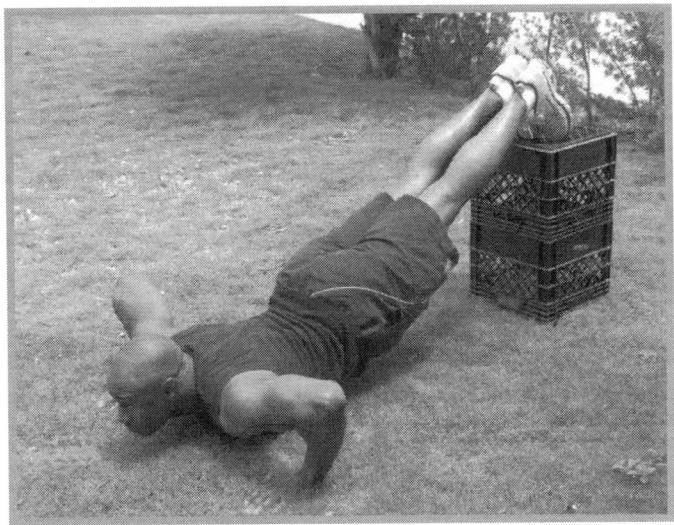

Finished Position

The Liederman Pushups.... This exercise is performed exactly as above. Hands on the floor, feet on a chair or stool at least 15 inches or more, the higher the stool the more the shoulders and upper chest work. Lower yourself as close to the ground as possible, then press back up again.

Across The Body Pulls Rear Delts (Contracted)

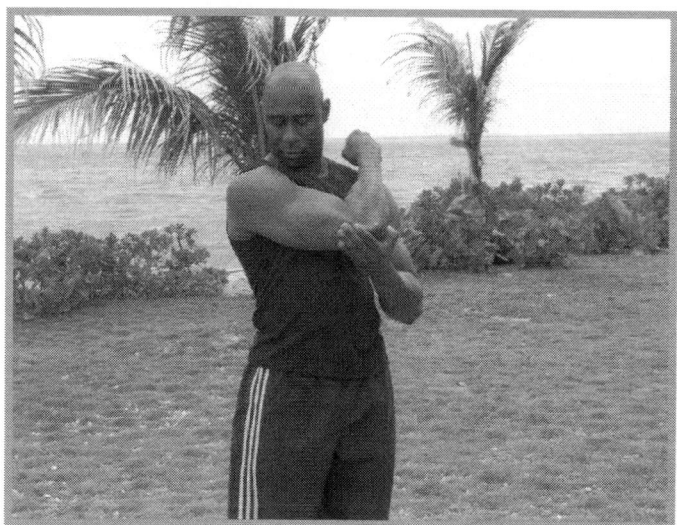

Start Position

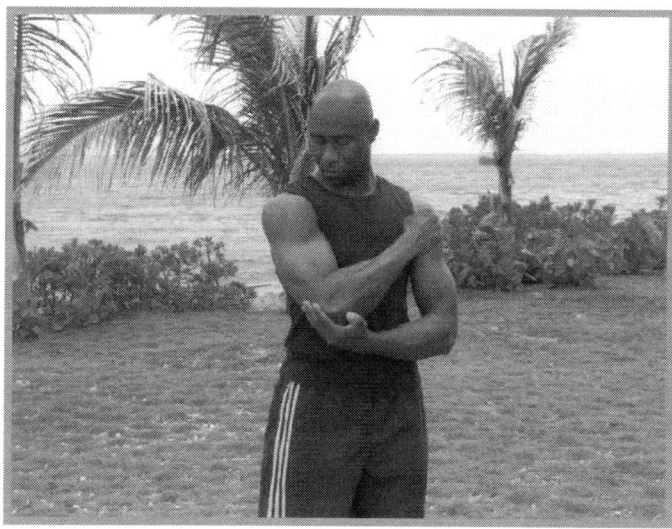

Finished Position

Grasp the right elbow as picture shows firmly with the left hand. Slowly force the right elbow downward and backward while resisting with the left hand. Repeat for reps, then switch arms. This add great strength and development to the (rear) back part of the shoulders, lats and mid-back. It's best to start with this exercise first for it's easily neglected in a muscle-building program. As they say, Out of site out of mind.

Resisted Forward Raises (Contracted)

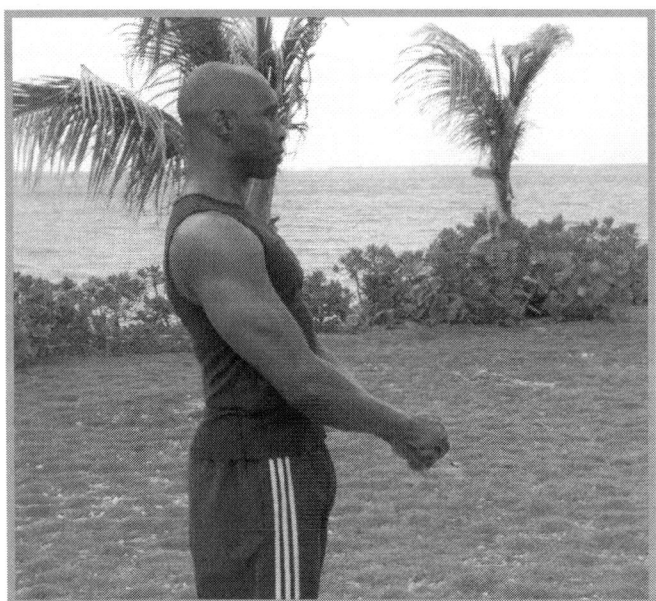

Start Position

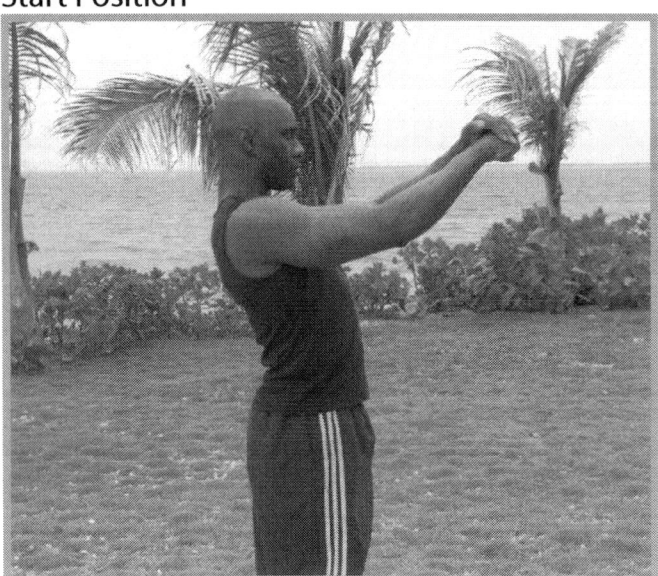

Finished Position

Grasp the right hand with the left in front of the body as shown. Gradually raise the arm forward against the resistance of the other hand. Repeat for reps. Then switch arms and continue. This works the Front shoulder muscles.

Side Lateral Raises (contracted)

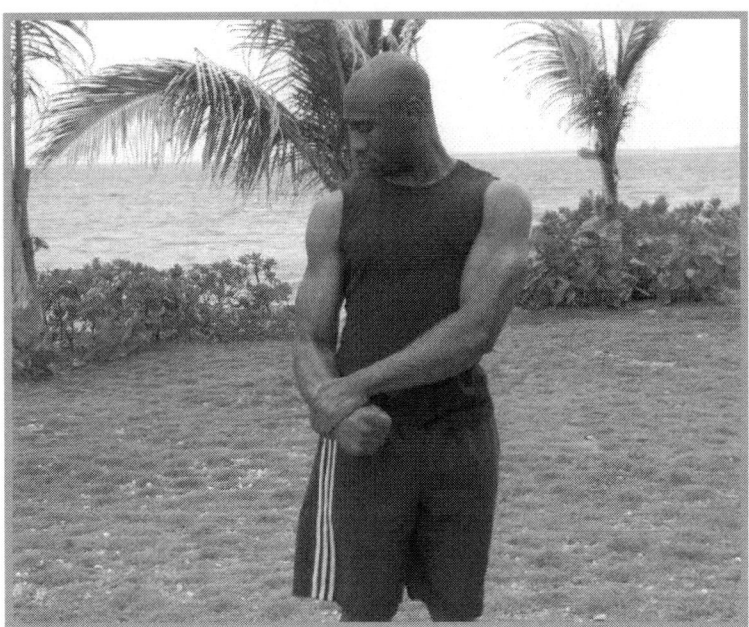
Start Position

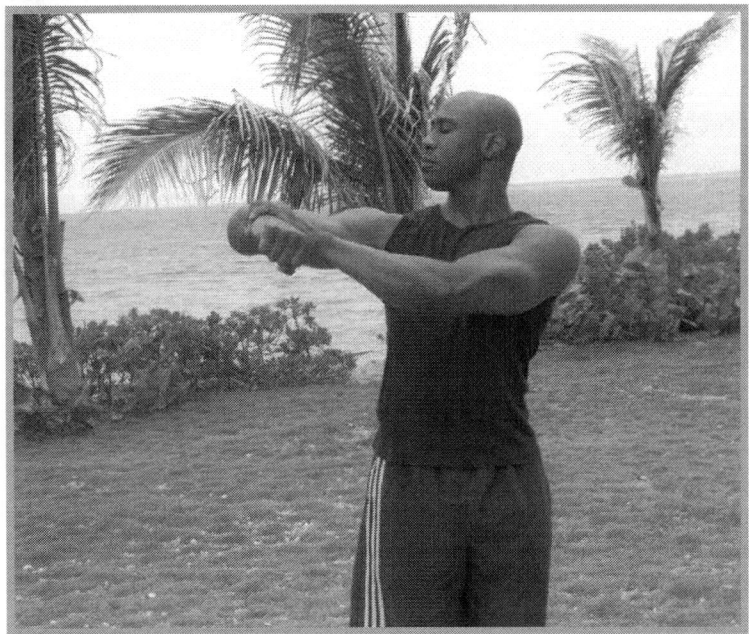
Finished Position

Maintain a bend on the right arm as shown. Grasp the wrist of the right arm and extend the arm out to the side while resisting with the left arm. This stimulate the side portion of the shoulders.

Across the Body Lateral Raises (Stretch and Contracted)

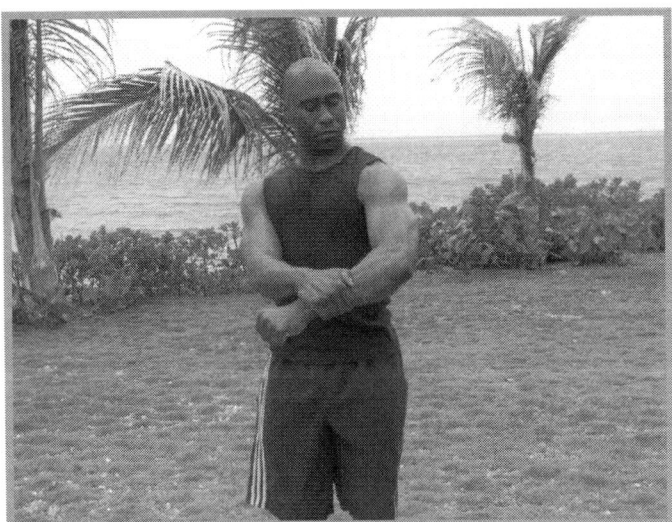

Start Position

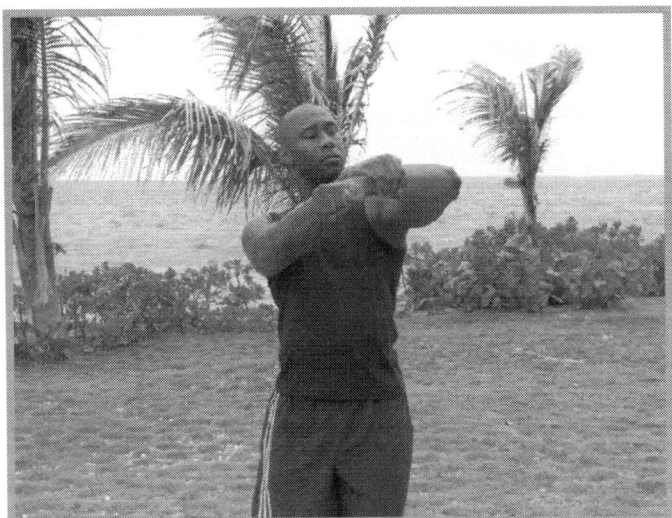

Finished Position

Grasp the left arm that is across the body as in the picture. Now raise the arm outwards towards the side contracted position resisting with the right arm. Perform desired reps then switch arms.

Resisted Shoulder Press (Basic and Contracted)

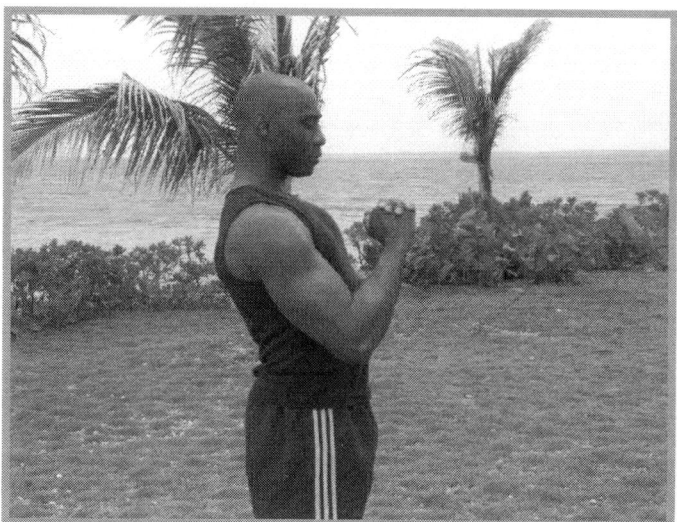

Start Position

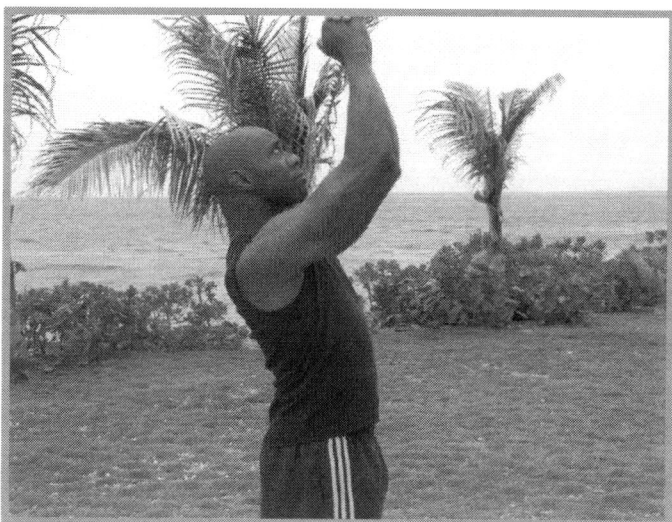

Finished Position

Place the left hand on-top of the right fist. Press the right arm upwards while resisting with the left hand. Reverse the movement at the top by pulling the left hand downwards while resisting with the right. Continue for reps then switch arms.

Resisted Upright Pulls (Basic and Contracted)

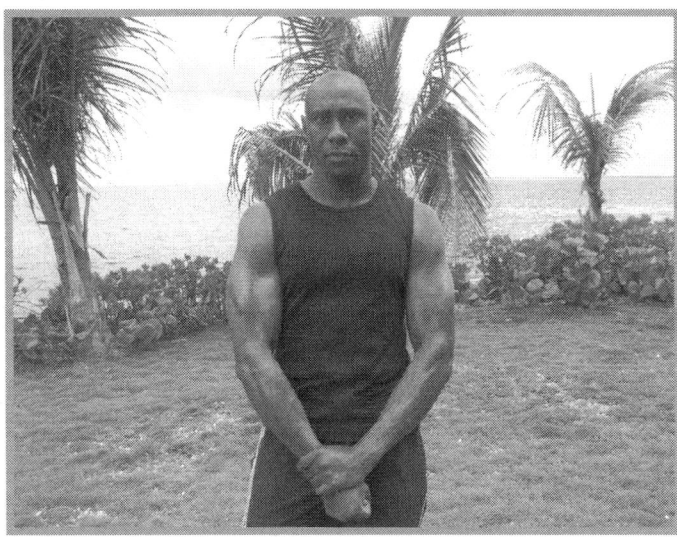

Start Position

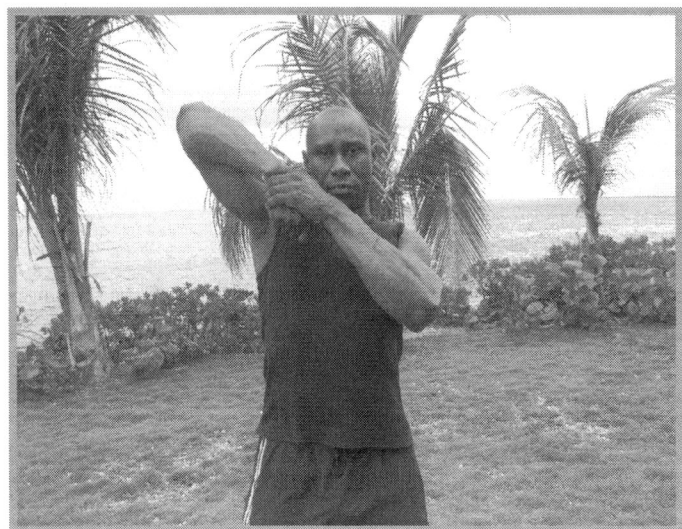

Finished Position

Hold onto the right wrist as shown above. Now pull the right arm upward while resisting with the left arm. Pull towards the ear, relax and repeat.

Bicep Exercises

Ok I've made a few changes to the original resisted curl to make it far more effective in building strength shape and muscle faster than before. At the very beginning while performing the original resisted curl gains were good but not great. Once I learned how to make the exercise harder and more efficient that's when my biceps and forearms really started to grow and take shape. It's all about efficiency in effort by changing this around to make it work better for you.

People are always looking at anyone that walk up that look a little fit or muscular, and what's the first thing they look at? The biceps and forearms. That's the first thing they see really. I've noticed it and all the people I've talked to about it have said so as well. It also helps when there's veins all around. What I've realized is that while I was developing or trying to develop my biceps and forearms my forearms got wider and was impressive when flexed , but my biceps looked narrow and when flexed flat looking. My biceps weren't as impressive hanging to my sides.

It wasn't wide enough. So I paid attention to the exercises that would make a difference and one of the lessons I learned is to change the way I did the regular Atlas curls at different angles and hand positioning. This made a difference with increasing the diameter of my biceps.

Now when I stood, I looked at my biceps in the mirror it's the inner part of the bicep that gives that width! Height is another thing that the long head on the outside and the muscle that's under the bicep needs to be developed as well.. the brachialis. Anyway, lets focus on what I did for the first phase then we'll break things down with the special Bicep and Tricep section later in this mini course. So here we go:

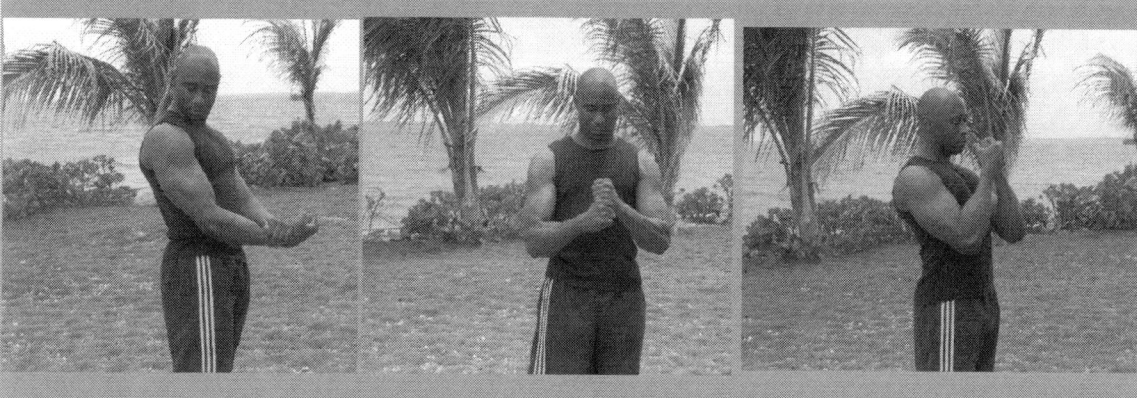

Now Let's look at the Muscle Sculpting Exercises.

Bicep Curl (Palm Up) (Basic)

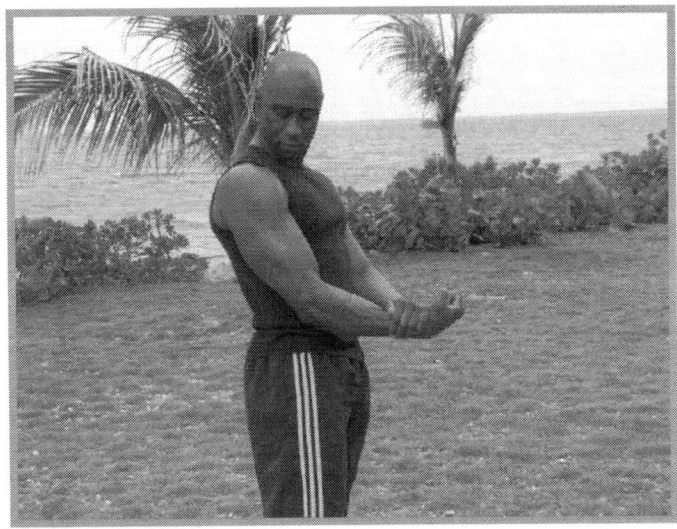

Start Position

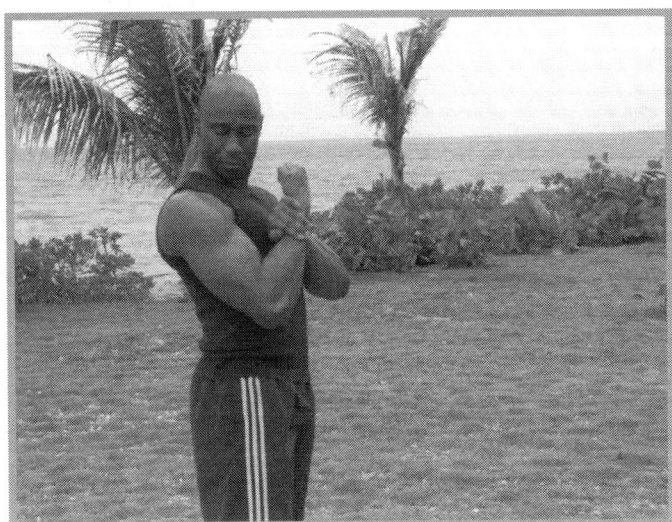

Finished Position

Grasp your right fist with the left hand. Pull the right arm upward towards the shoulder while resisting with the left hand. At the shoulder, reverse the exercise by pushing the left arm downwards resisting with the right. Continue for reps then switch arms.

Another Variation Palm Up Curls (Basic)

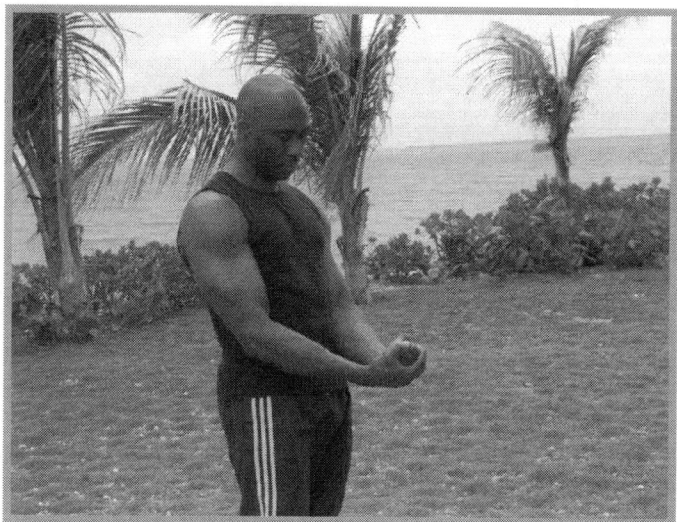
Start Position

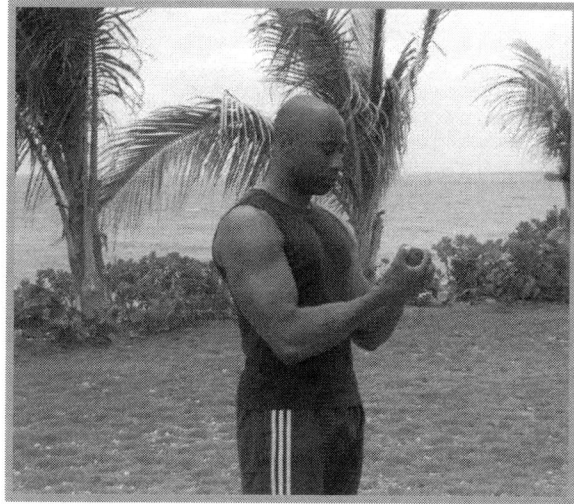
Mid-Point

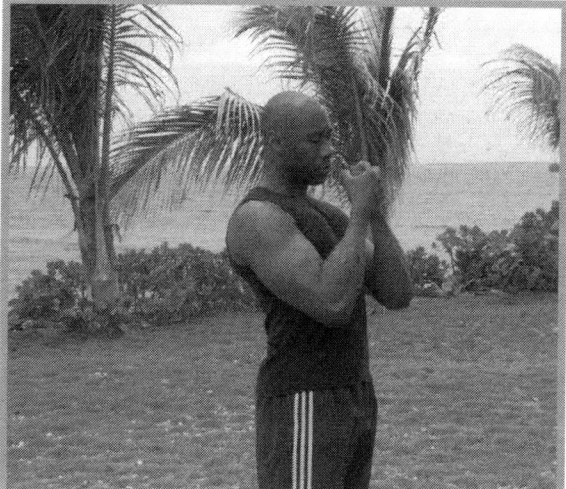
Finished Position

This is another version of the palm up curl that's far efficient than the original version. This time place the left hand inside of the right hand. Now pull the right hand up towards the chest resisting with the left hand. Reverse the exercise at the top by pushing the left hand down resisting with the right for reps, then switch arms. This gives the biceps Awesome leverage for a greater bicep contraction.

Reverse Bicep/Forearm Curls

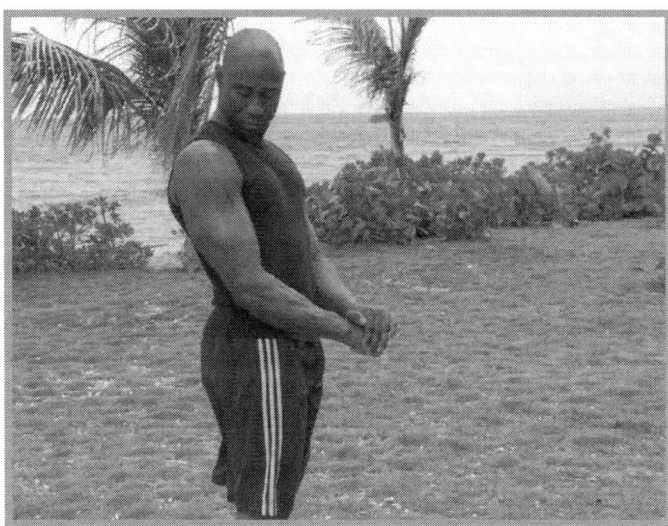

Start Position

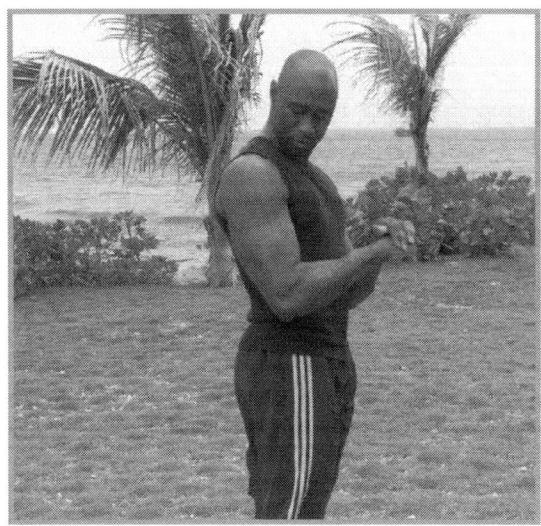

Mid-Point

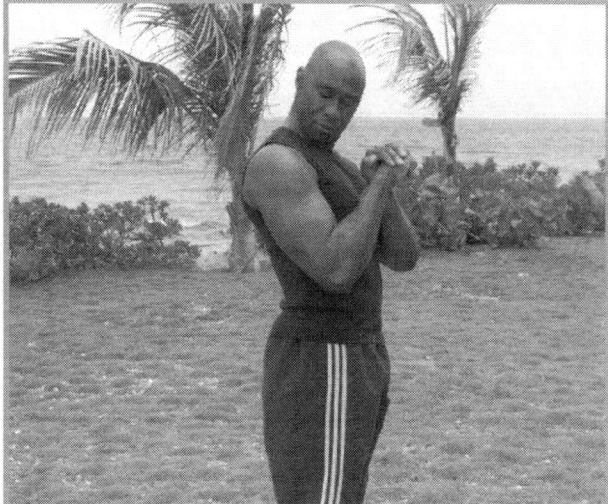

Finished Position

This is the Grand-Daddy of all exercises. A Great bicep/forearm widener. Place the left hand on top of the right fist. Now pull the right arm upwards while resisting with the left hand. At the shoulder reverse the exercise by pushing the left arm downwards resisting with the right hand. Repeat for reps then switch arms.

Hammer Curls (Basic)

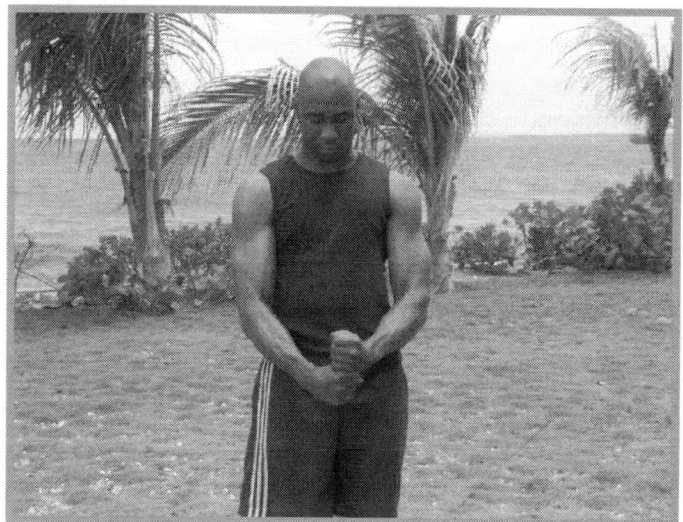

Start Position

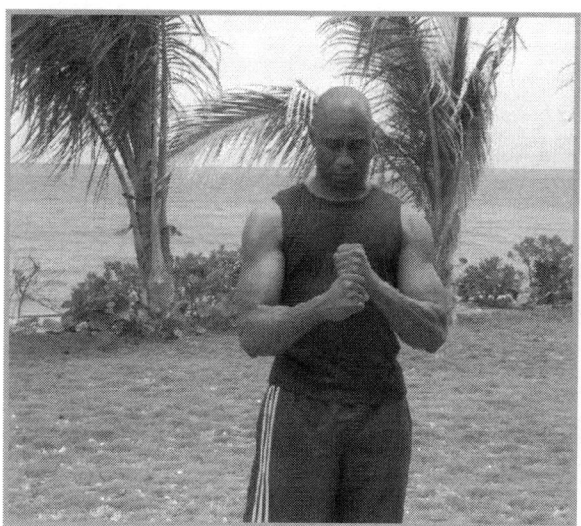

Mid- Point

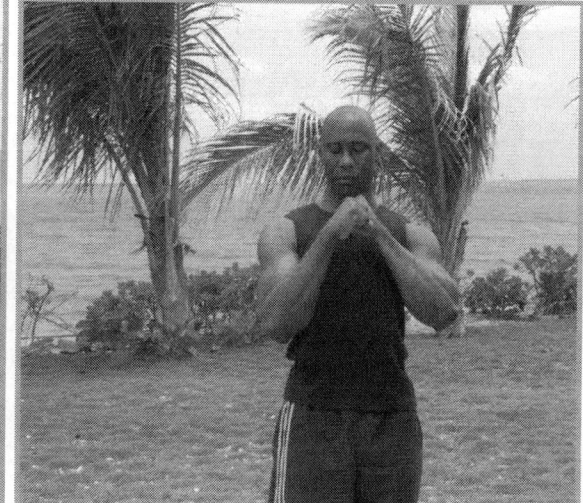

Finished Position

Another great Bicep/Forearm combo. Place the wrists as shown in the picture above. Now pull with the right hand or bottom hand upwards to the chest while resisting with the top hand. At upper chest level reverse the exercise by pressing the top wrist down and resisting with the bottom wrist. Repeat for reps then switch arms.

Over-Head Curls (contracted)

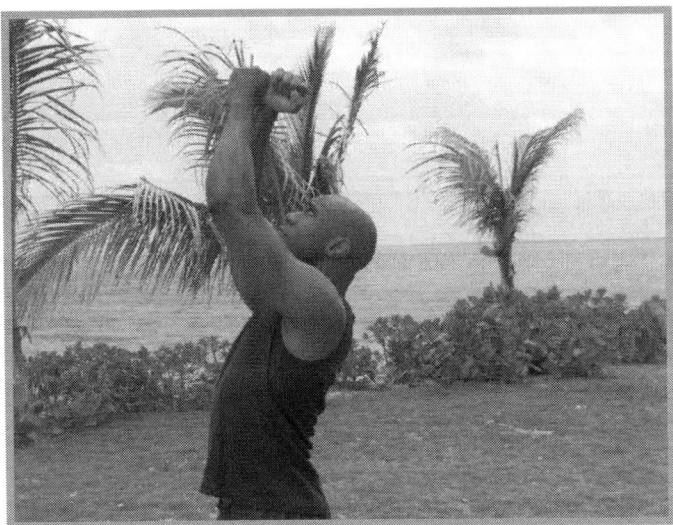

Start Position

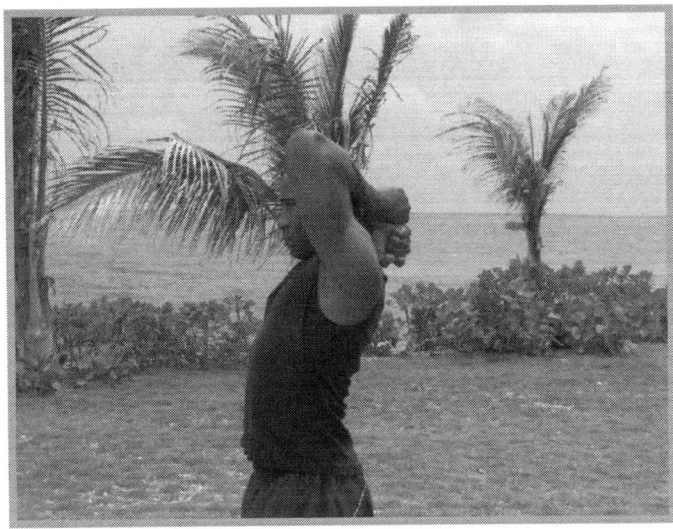

Finished Position

This exercise stimulates the long head of the biceps increasing the bicep height and fullness. Place the hands in fists as shown. Now pull the top hand downwards while resisting with the bottom. Reverse the exercise by pressing the bottom hand upwards and resisting with the top. Use a moderate tension due to elbow sensitivity on this over head position.

Concentration Curls (contracted)

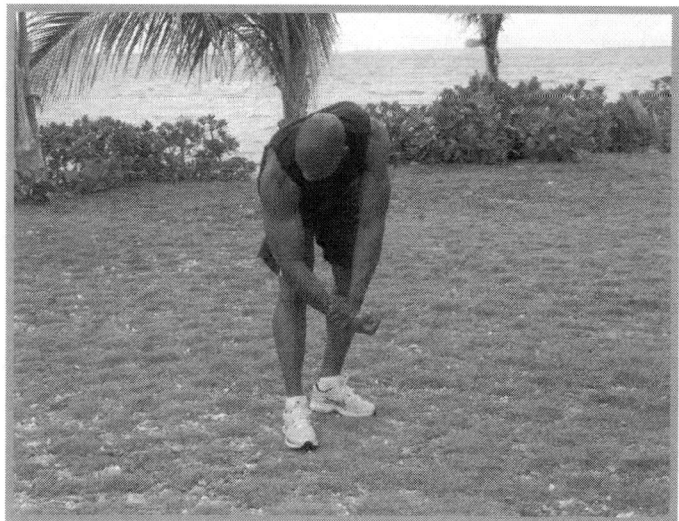

Start Position

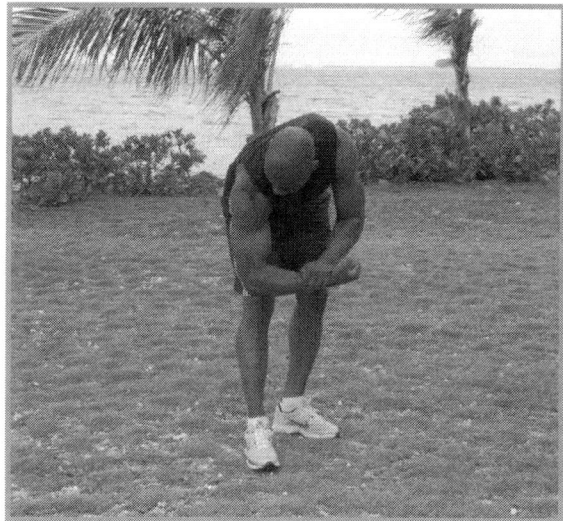

Mid-Point

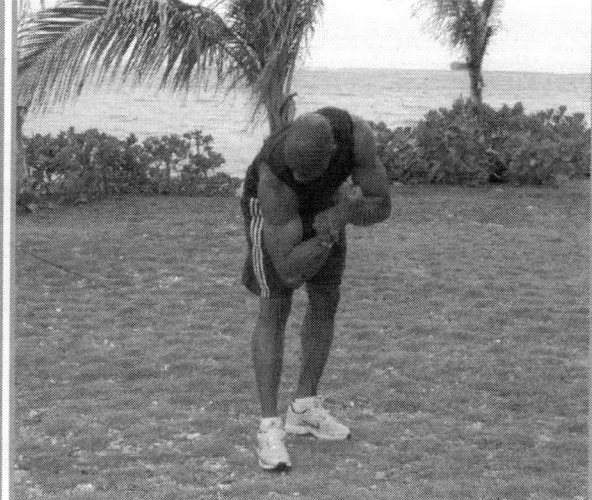

Finished Position

This is a great bicep finisher move. Peak contraction to hit that long head again. As pictured in start position hold onto the right wrist with left hand and pull the right arm towards the face while resisting with the left hand. Now reverse the exercise by pushing the left arm down and resisting with the right. Complete your reps then switch arms and repeat movement.

Tricep Exercises

The triceps long head is the largest part of the tricep musculature. It's responsible for the most tricep size. The tricep is broken into 3 muscle-heads. Lateral (outer head), Long Head (inside muscle), and the Middle or medial head. (middle muscle). The tricep is easily developed due to dips, pushups and a variety of self resistance type exercises. The self resistance exercises are geared to stimulate the tricep throughout the full range motion through 3 separate ranges of push.

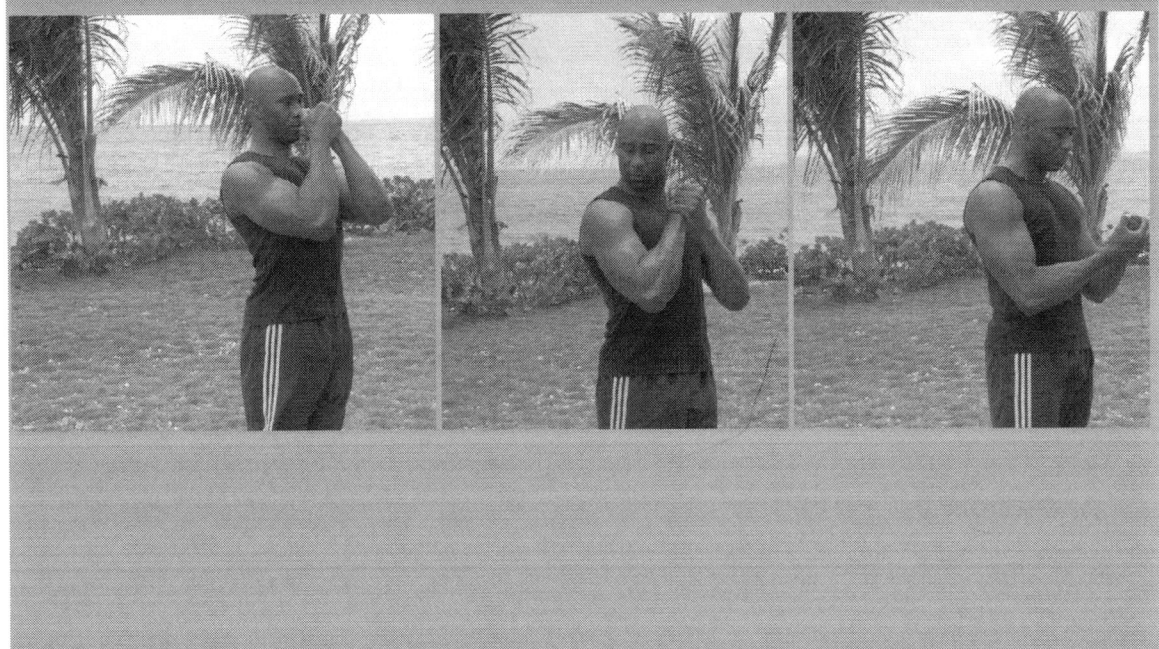

Forward Tricep Press (Basic)

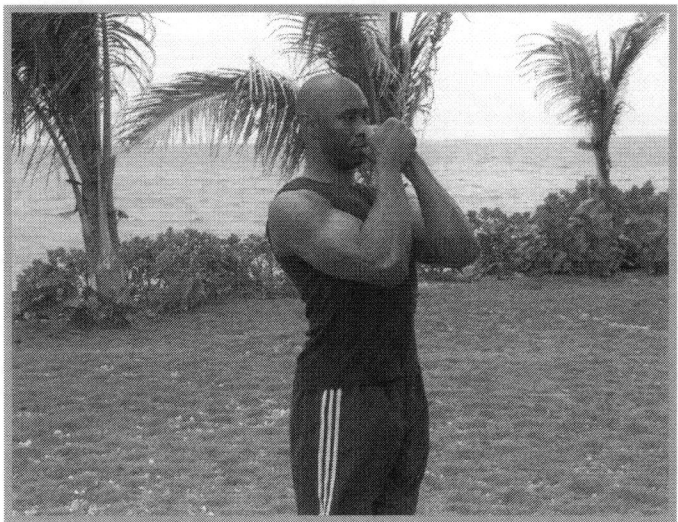

Start Position

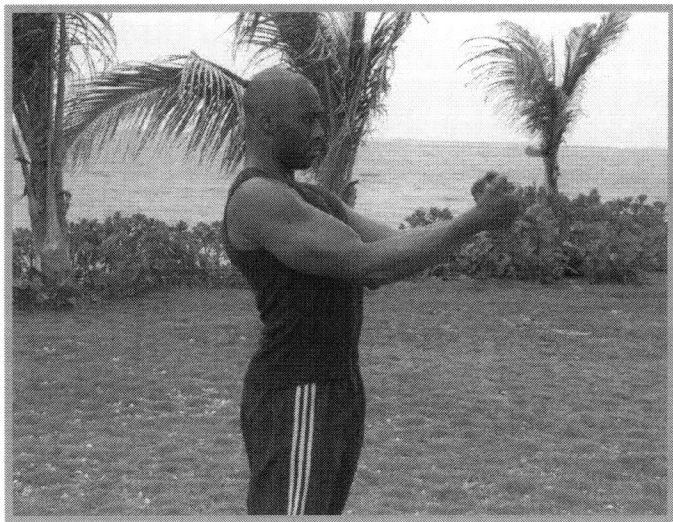

Finished Position

Place the left fist in the right hand. Now push the left hand forward while resisting with the right hand. At the finished position reverse the movement by pulling the right hand towards you resisting with the left.

Tricep Pressdown (contracted)

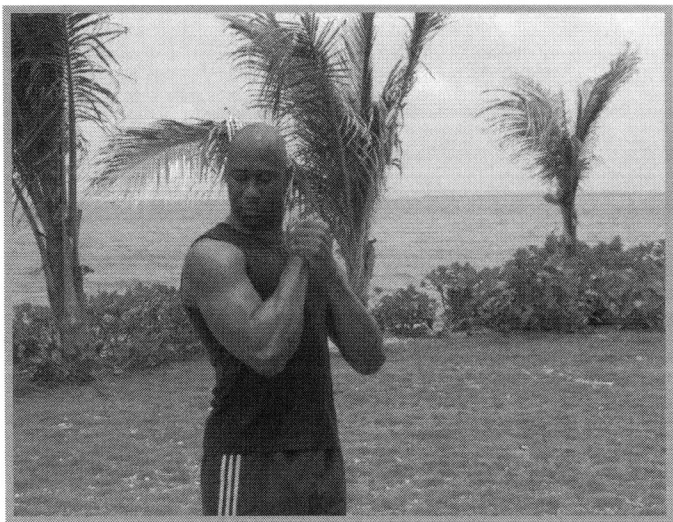

Start Position

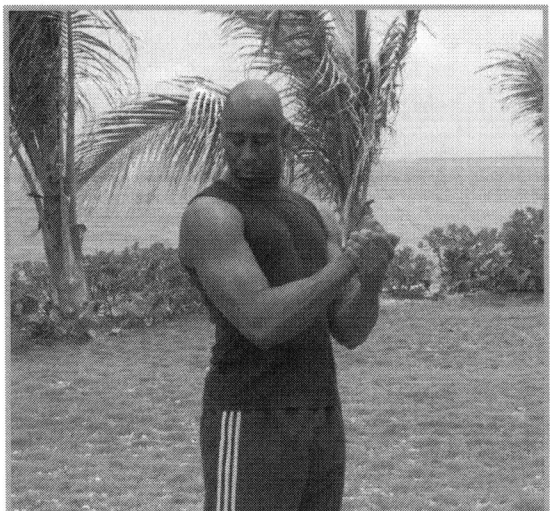

Mid-Point

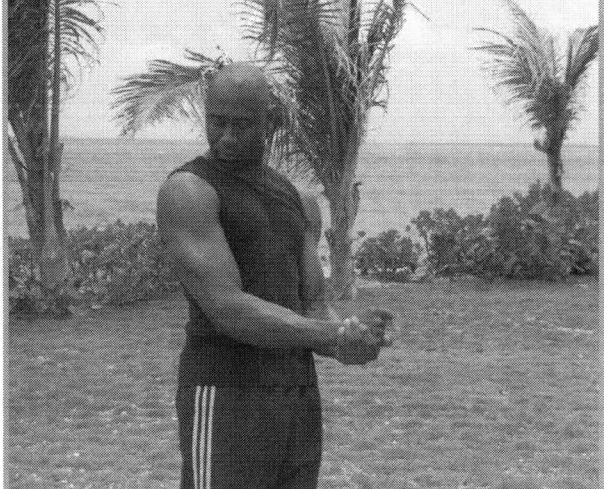

Finished Position

Make a fist with the right hand and place it in the left. Now press the right hand downwards while resisting with the left hand. Repeat desired reps then switch arms.

Over Head Tricep Press (stretch, contracted)

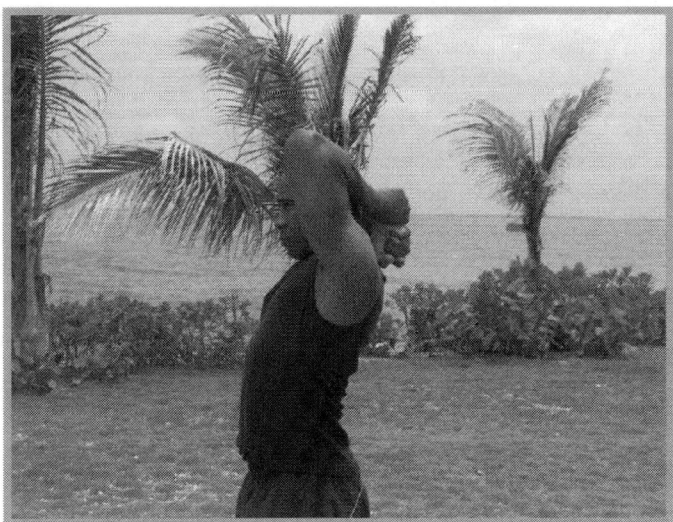

Start Position

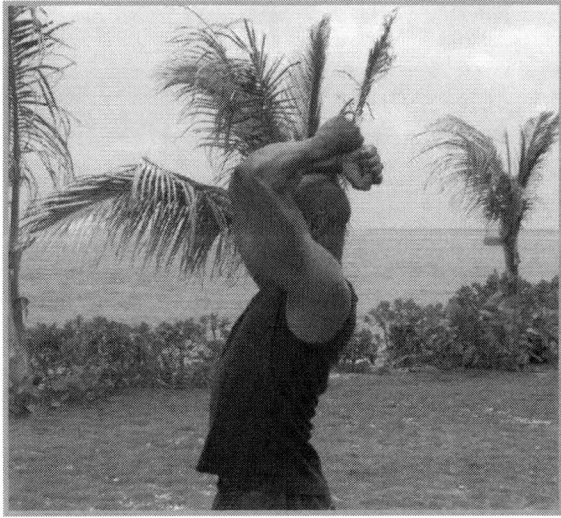

Mid-Point

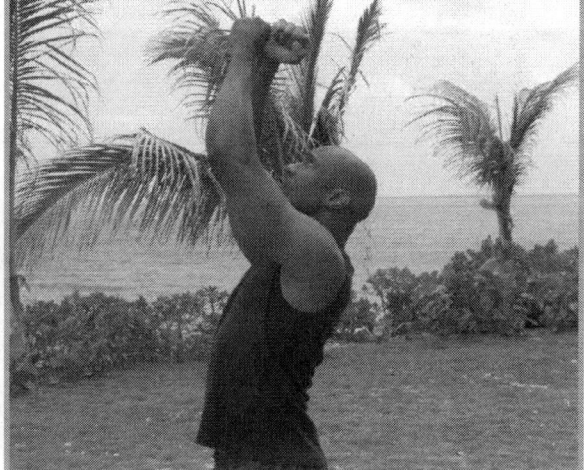

Finished Position

Make a fist with both hands place it behind your neck. Now press the bottom fist upward while resisting with the top fist. At the top reverse the exercise by pushing downwards with the top fist while resisting with the bottom fist. Use a light to moderate tension due to the tricep tendons being quite sensitive at that position.

Decline Tricep Extensions (Basic)

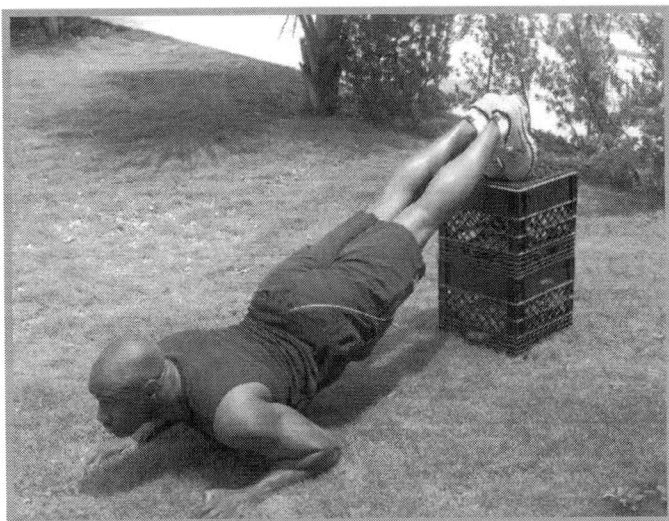

Start Position

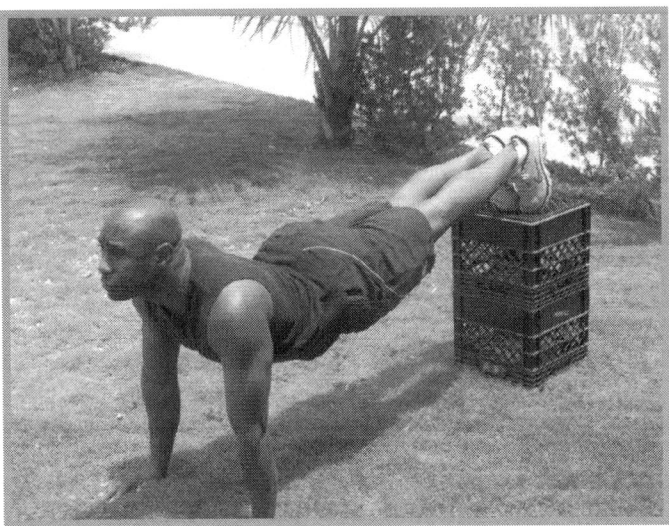

Finished Position

Place your feet on a chair or box as shown in the picture. Place your hands and lower-arms on the floor and slowly press the arm straight out with a slight bend to the elbows. This exercise stimulates the outer head (lateral) muscle of the triceps.

Palm Up Tricep Press Down (contracted)

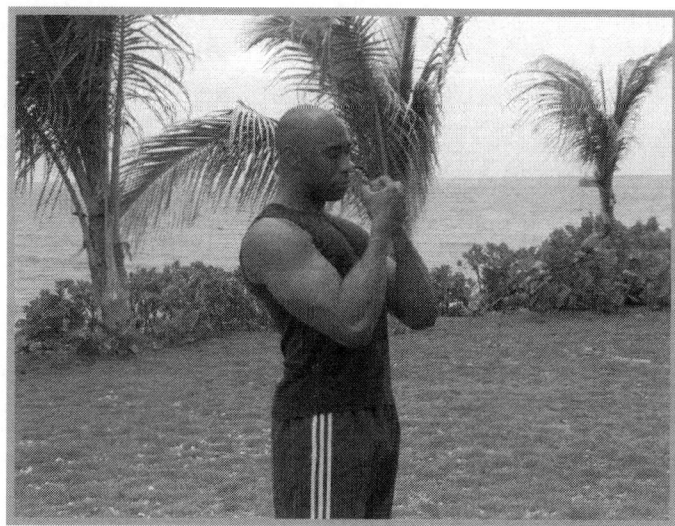

Start Position

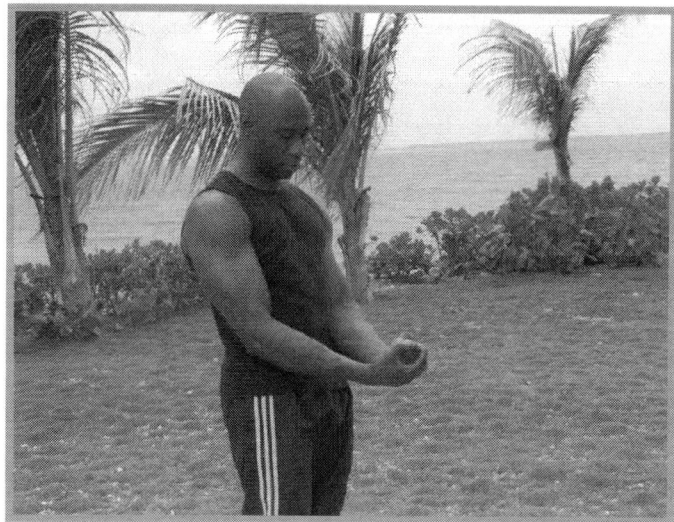

Finished Position

Place the left fist palm up in the right hand. Now press the left hand downwards resisting with the right hand. Relax and repeat movement.

Forearms

Powerful forearms just like upper arms command respect! This muscle needs to be balanced with the upper arm. Last thing you want are forearms that look weak with powerful upper-arms. So, here's a number of exercises to increase the griping strength, and overall musculature of the lower arm, connective tissues of the wrists and increases and strengthens the grip. The brachialis muscle that runs under the biceps and into the forearm, is the one muscle that's strongly targeted here. Resisted hammer curls and reverse curls gets the job done with a bicep effect as a tag-on! So these two exercises are the best efficient (basic) forearm-bicep exercises. These two exercises were covered earlier in our bicep exercises. So here we go again.

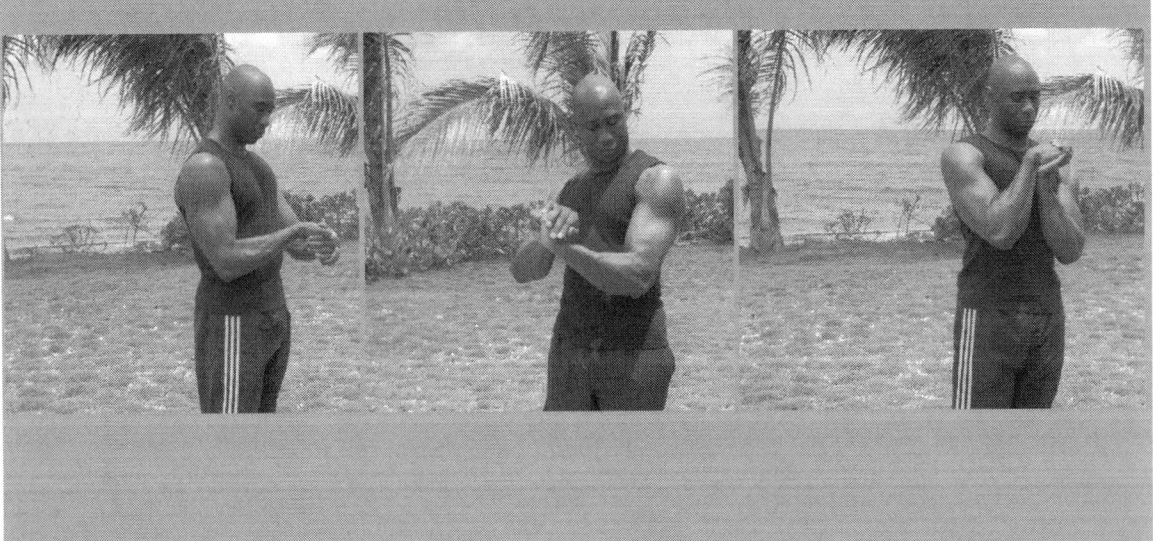

Palm Up Wrist Curls

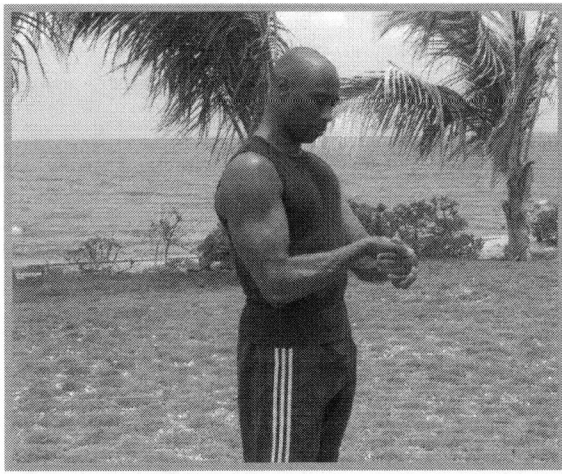
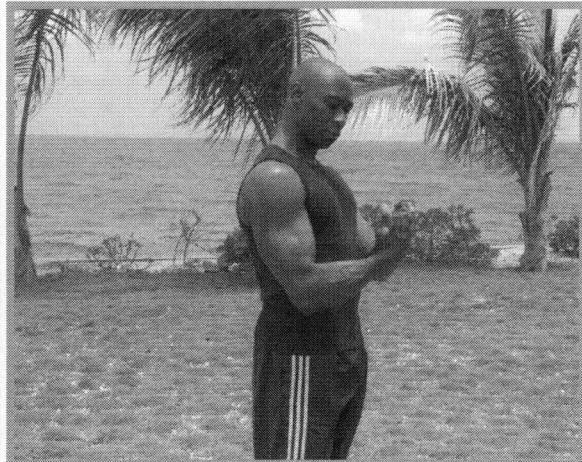

Start Position   Finished Position

As pictured extend the right wrist backwards placing the left hand pressed against. Now Flex the right wrist upwards while resisting with the left hand. Practice till tired or desired reps are done then switch hands and repeat.

Reverse Palm Down Wrist Curls

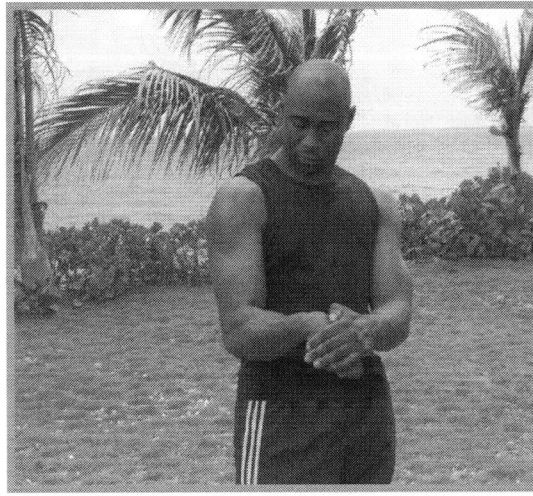

Start Position   Finished Position

Same as before but this time the palm in pressed down. Resist with the opposite hand for reps then reverse hands.

Reverse Curls and Hammer Curls

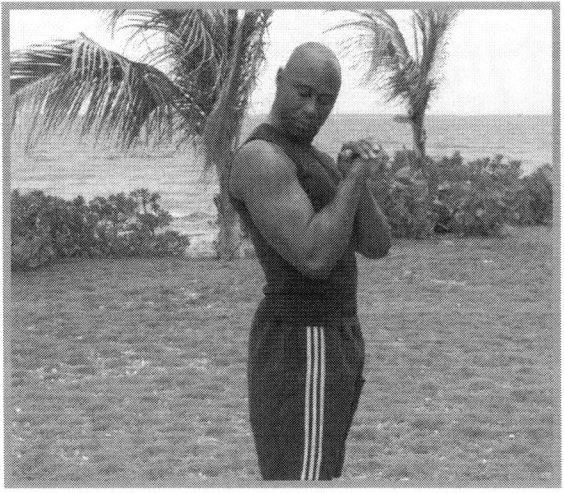 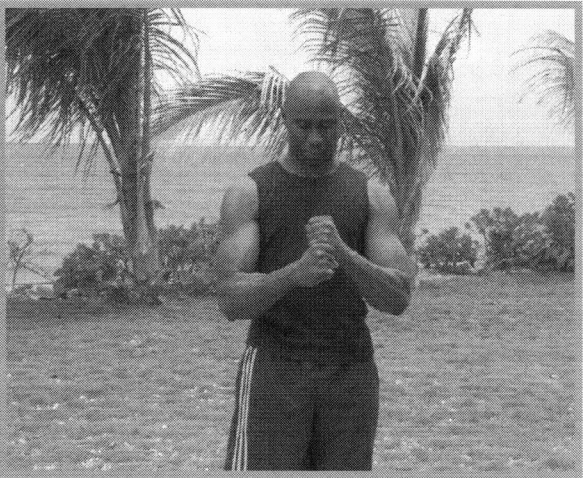

The forearms wonuld not be complete without hitting the brachialis muscle that runs under the biceps. It is a great Bicep/Forearm combo.

Forearm Presses

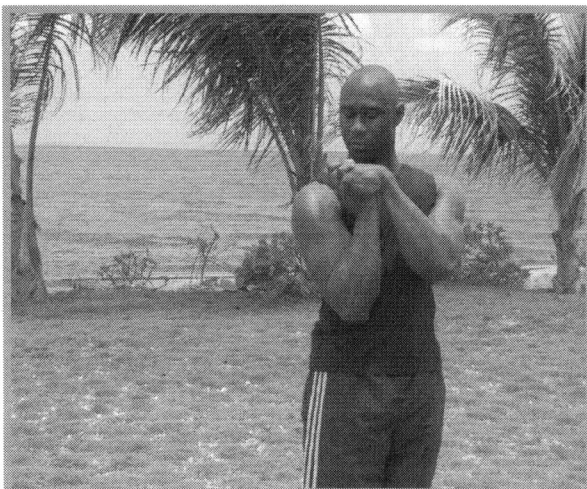 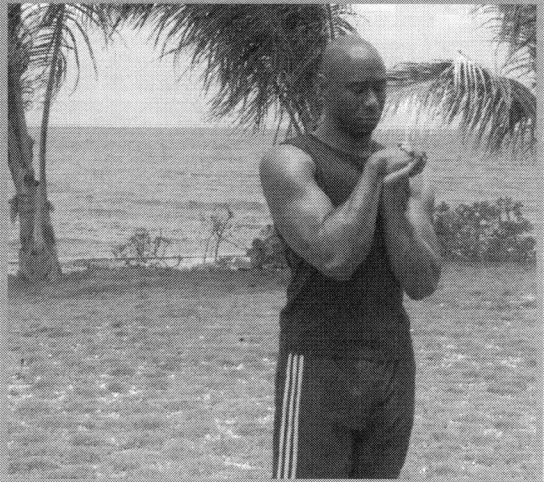

Start Position   Finished Position

Perform this exercise as pictured by pressing to one side then the other while resisting with the opposite hand.

Thigh & Hamstrings

Ok let's focus on the Powerful thighs and hamstring development exercises. Developing strength and power is what every athlete as well as every person wants. How do we achieve that? Let's start from the very top: Regular Squats the King of All Lower-Body exercises stimulate everything! Thighs, Hips, Hamstrings, Inner Thighs and Glutes (butt). Followed by Leg extensions, and leg curls we are talking maximum efficiency. Multi-Joint exercises that stimulate the important hips, thighs and glutes is all we need. Let's get on with it..

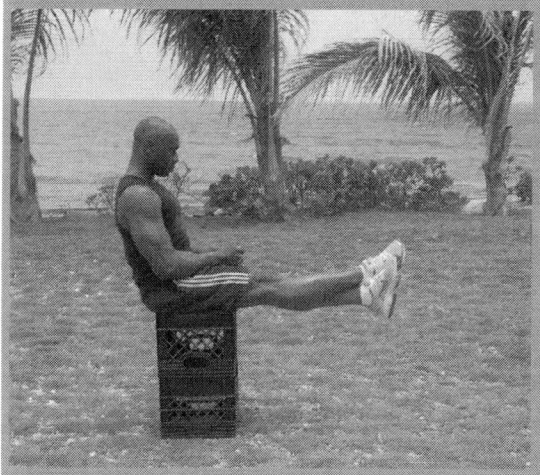
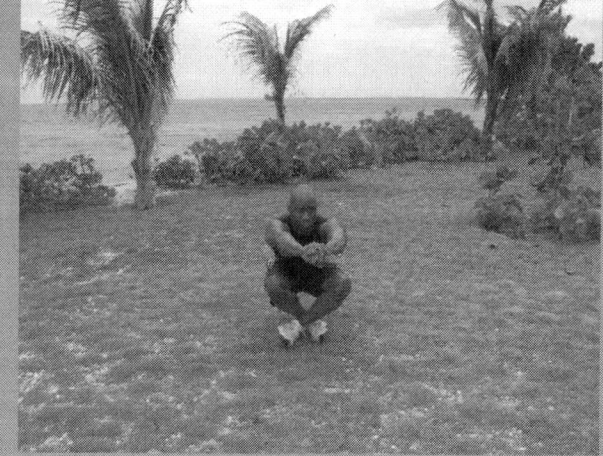

Regular Squats

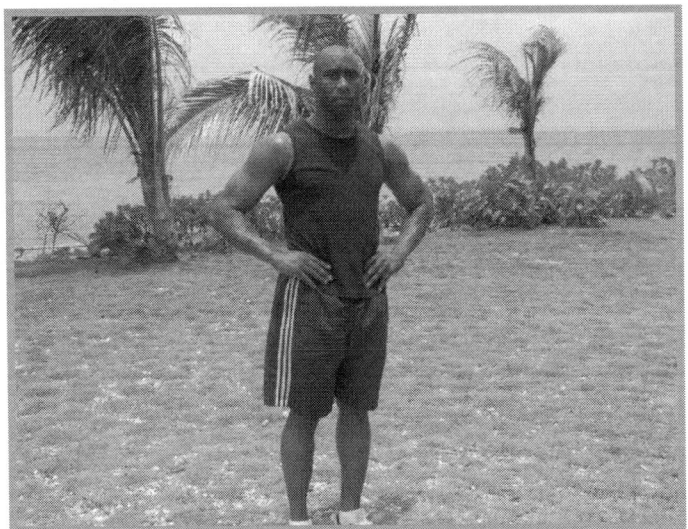

Start Position

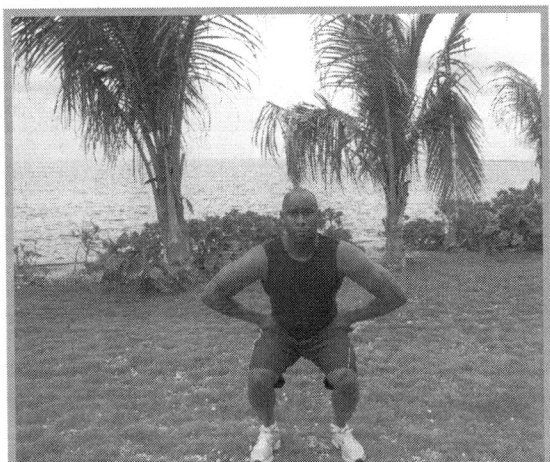

Mid-Point

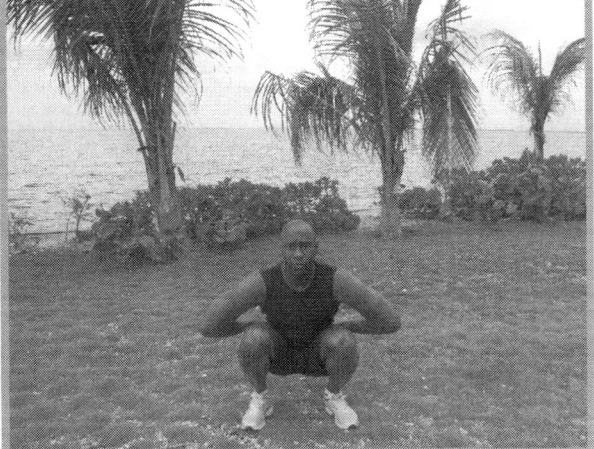

Finished Position

This is the easiest of body-weight exercises. Start off as the start position shows then lower yourself under control to the finished position. Now reverse the movement by coming up again to the start position. Continue for desired reps. Do Not Bounce.

Crossed Feet Squats

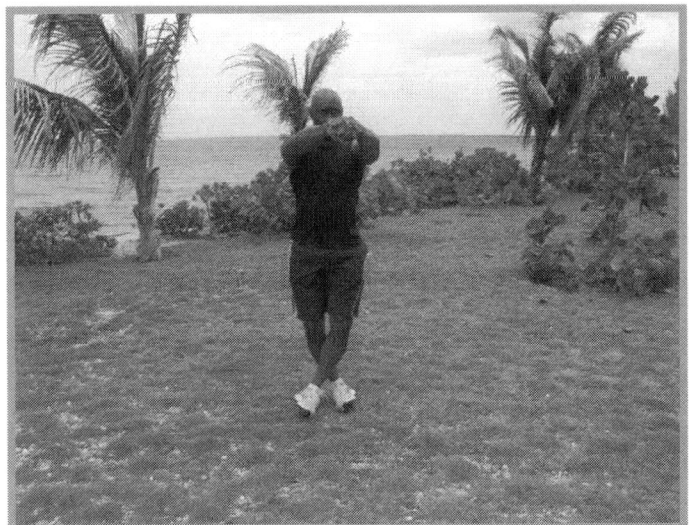

Start Position

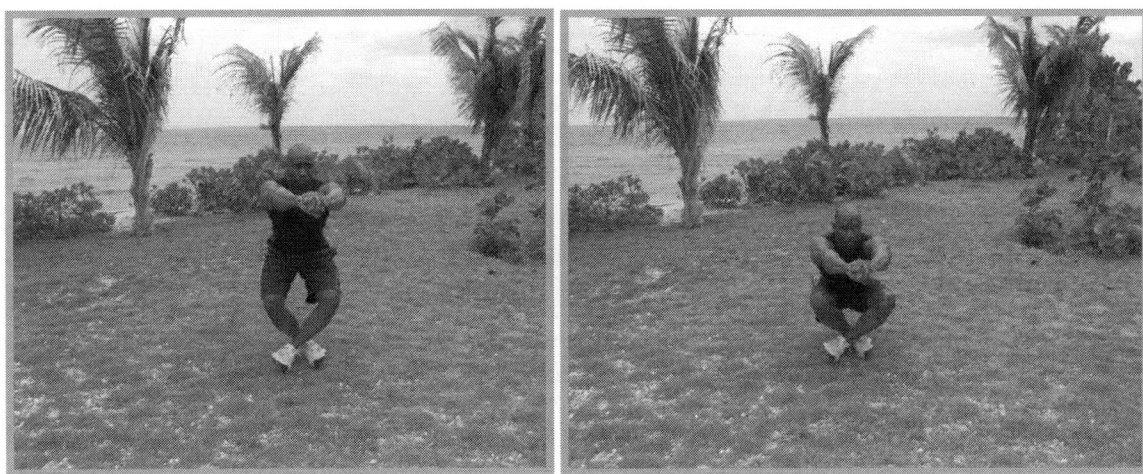

Mid-Point   Finished Position

Another excellent exercise for the overall thigh and hamstrings. Start off as shown in the starting position with feet crossed. Slowly under control lower yourself to the finished position No Bouncing. One second pause then reverse the movement to the starting position. This exercise may be difficult at first but keep practicing and as night follows day it gets easier.

Resisted Leg Extensions

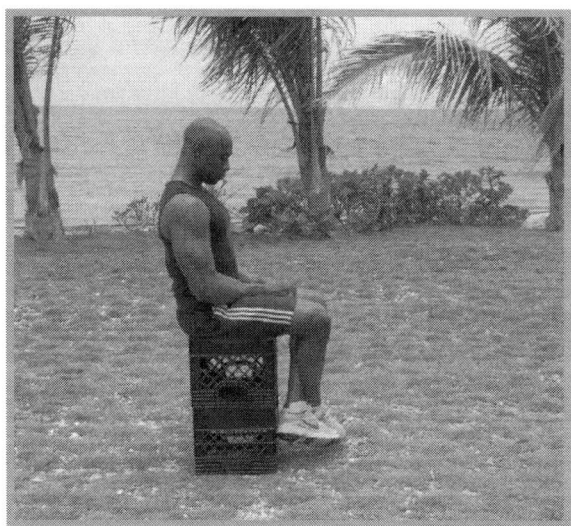

Start Position

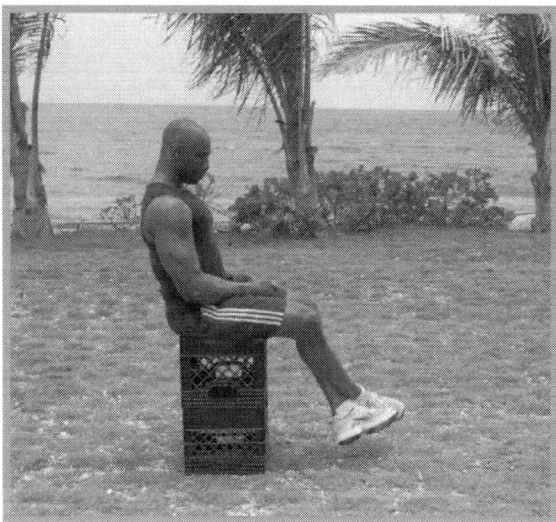

Mid-Point

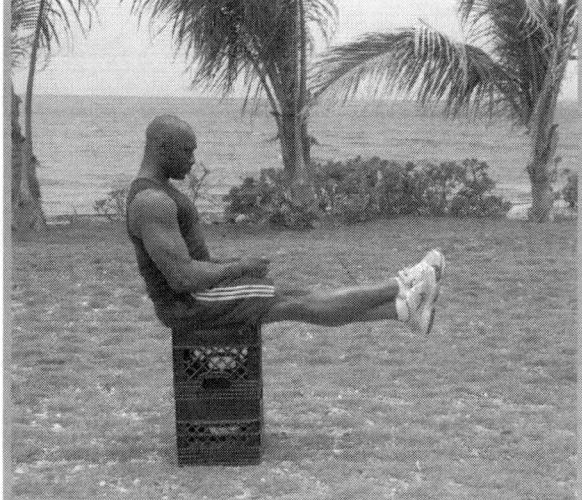

Finished Position

While seated on a chair, box or stool, place the right leg over the left as shown in the picture, and extend the left leg outwards resisting with the right. At the top reverse the movement by pulling down the right while resisting with the left.

Hamstring Resisted Leg Curl

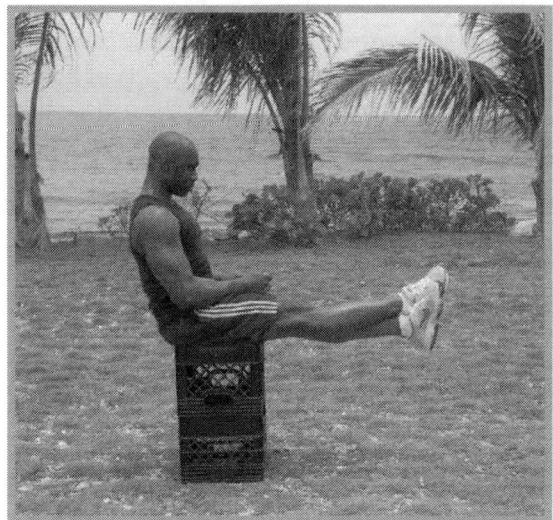

Start Position

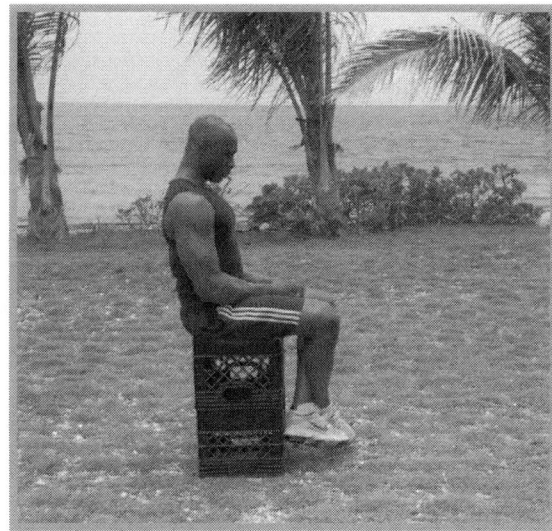

Finished Position

Just like the exercise above but the reverse. At the start position pull the top leg down only resisting with the bottom leg. Repeat for reps.

Resisted Lying Leg Curls

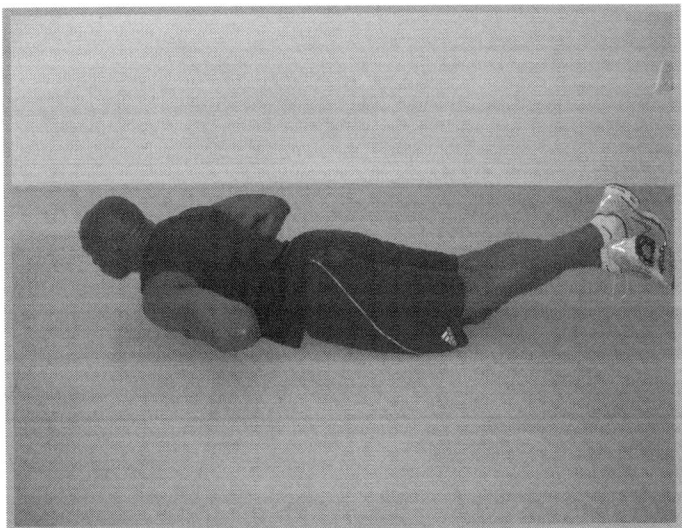

Start Position

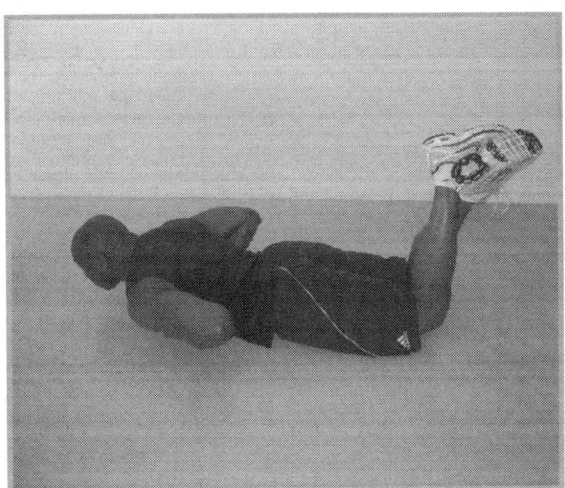

Mid-Point

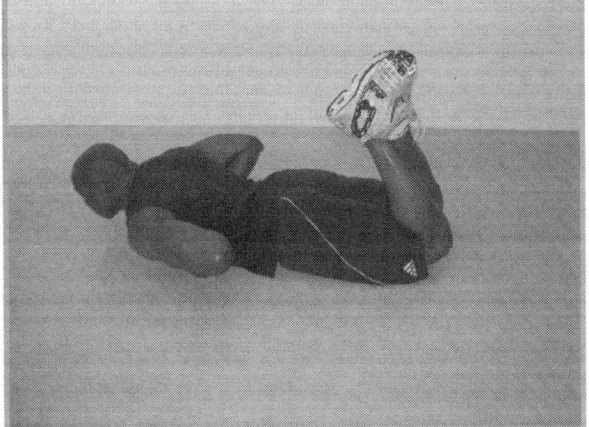

Finished Position

While on the stomach on the floor place the left leg over the right as shown, Now pull the right leg upwards towards you while resisting with the left leg. Pull on the Up phase only. Repeat for reps then switch legs.

Calve Training

Now calf growth due to the dense layers of the muscles itself is quite stubborn! So my results within this department wasn't the best. However, I've learned a few things. In order for my calves to improve various steps had to be taken into consideration. I did loads of high reps daily but lost the true meaning of building muscle within this area. In order to add muscle onto those it's best to really focus on how you're doing the exercises and what rep range you're using for ultimate muscle-building stimulation, which I'll explain in a moment).

Here they are:
Stretch: You achieve this position at the bottom of any calf exercise—calves stretched off a high block. It's important to get that stretch to force the calves to contract at it's maximum!

HIGH REPS. As I've said earlier the calve is one dense muscle. The majority of these calf fibers are Endurance Oriented Fibers. Because it's used daily. You contract these muscles all day by walking. So they need to be taxed a certain way. The best way to target the calves are with reps that hit the range between 30 to 35 reps per set. Tension times are increased for your straight sets of calf work and should be about one minute or more, to efficiently hit the dense fibers effectively.

FEEL. As with any muscle group you must pay attention to the feel and focus on the muscle at hand. It is important to avoid bouncing and fast reps. Rep speed is also important. Three seconds up and the same speed for the down portion is about right. But feel is the most important element here.

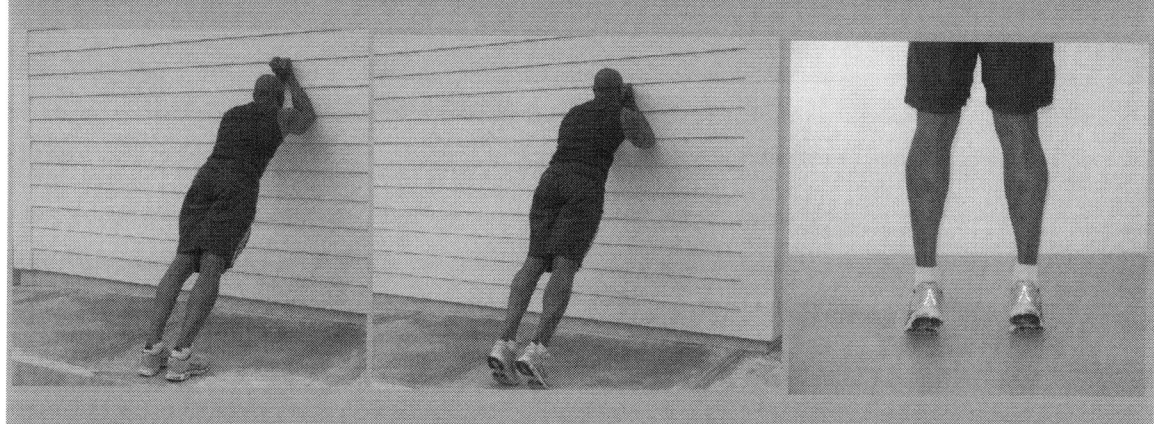

Another key to maximizing calf development and to increase the stress is to maintain the tension on the calve muscles. By not coming all the way up to full contraction this maintains constant tension on the muscle and increases blood blockage. This will indeed increase growth stimulation, capillary development and muscle overload and what about the bottom range?

This is just as important. It's important to get a max stretch at the bottom of the movement. This really pre-stretches the muscles to fire more efficiently due to the powerful stretch that loosens up the fibers, which produces additional growth.

More Calf-Growing Details

Now guys I don't have genetically superior calve development. Well not yet anyway.. still working on it, according to my wife. After my experiment I added a component that was never done for my calves effectively, but last year my calves got even better than the year before with less work per set. They looked almost two inches bigger. It didn't make sense really. So I introduced a number of techniques and stress methods into my calve workouts for the first time To see the effects of it all. Lo and behold my calves responded far better to the stress methods.

After all, my calves looked much better with more size and shape and increased vascularity more naturally. Now I'm not blessed with inner-calf flare. So seeing that the methods increased that fact I loved it to the max. By doubling up on the key contracted point of the movement with mini reps at the end of my full reps made the set far more intense. That's only one method I did. You will see more in later chapters in the routine sections.

Standing Cave Raises (stretch and contracted)

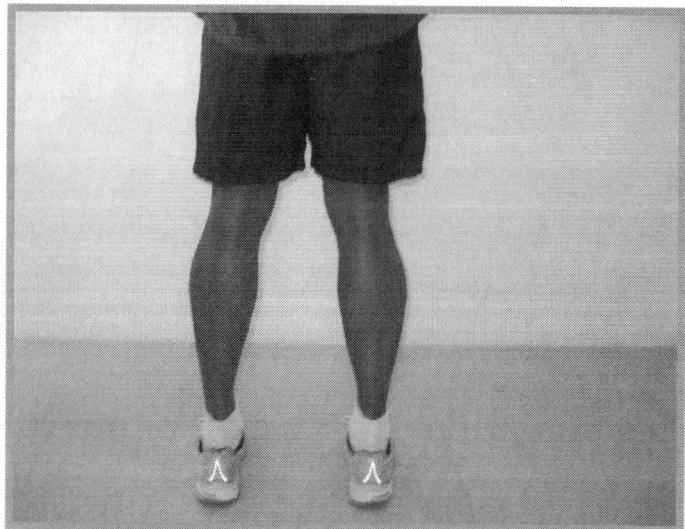

Start Position

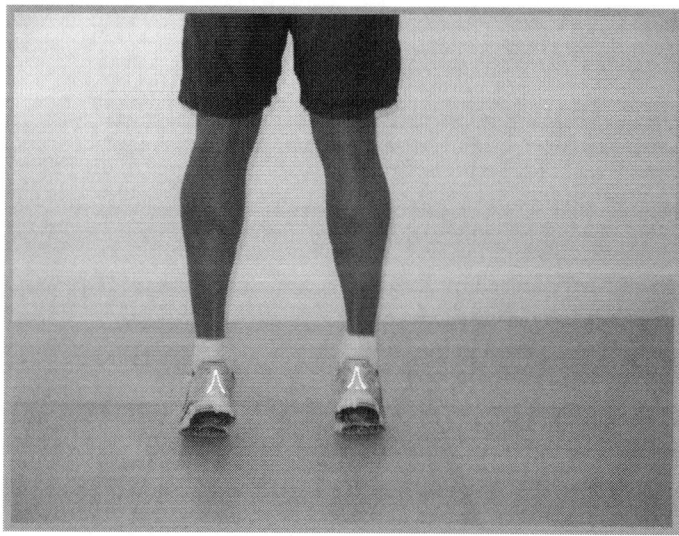

Finished Position

This exercise can be done on the stairs or block. Start as shown and go up and down contracting the calves at the top of the movement. If on stairs, extend the heels as low as you can to really pre-stretch the calves, then press upwards into the contracted position. (finished position)

Slanted Pre-Stretch Calve Raises

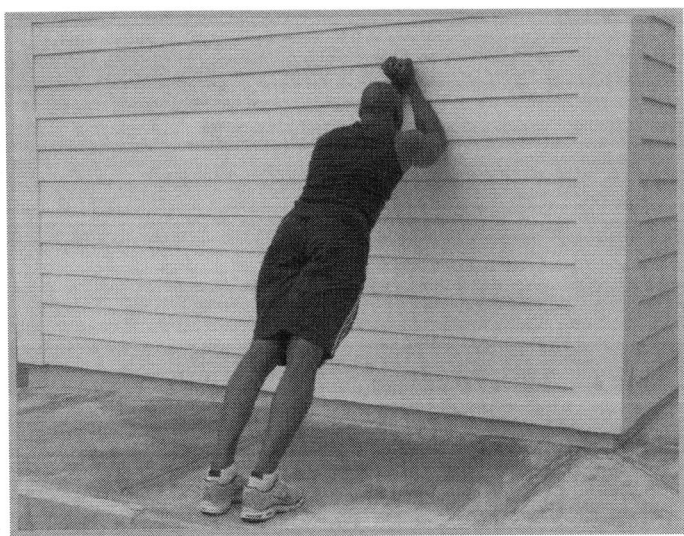

Start Position

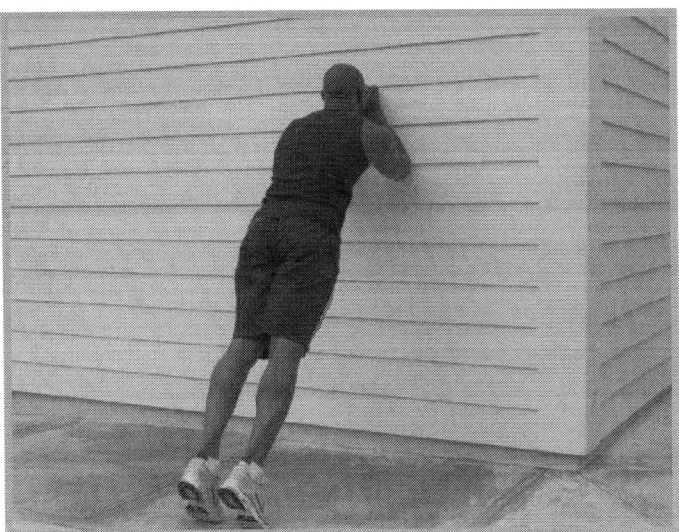

Finished Position

Stand at least 30 inches away from the wall, or position yourself as shown but make sure the calves are well stretched. Start off as shown in the picture start position. Press straight up on the toes then lower. This is as awesome calve stretch exercise. Perform this exercise until the calves are well tired. This stimulates the entire calve.

Abdominal Training

Abdominal Training are endurance type fiber muscles. Very much like forearms and calve muscles. Which means they need longer tension times and high rep ranges to benefit from training. Muscle Makeup. The abdominal muscles are just that—muscles. It's one sheet of muscles with tendons dividing the muscles into blocks. So, it isn't upper and lower it's one sheet. Each is made up of the same types of fibers as your biceps, chest and back; however, as I mentioned, many of the fibers in the abs are more endurance oriented and require higher reps to reach full development. The main abdominal muscle that one need to be concerned with, is the rectus abdominis, (front area) this isn't a bunch of knotted musles, as it appears to be, but rather a sheet-type muscle that runs from the bottom of your rib cage and attaches to your pelvis. As I've said earlier, The ripples are actually caused by tendons running horizontally and vertically. Throughout the entire length that cause the block type muscle separation you see.

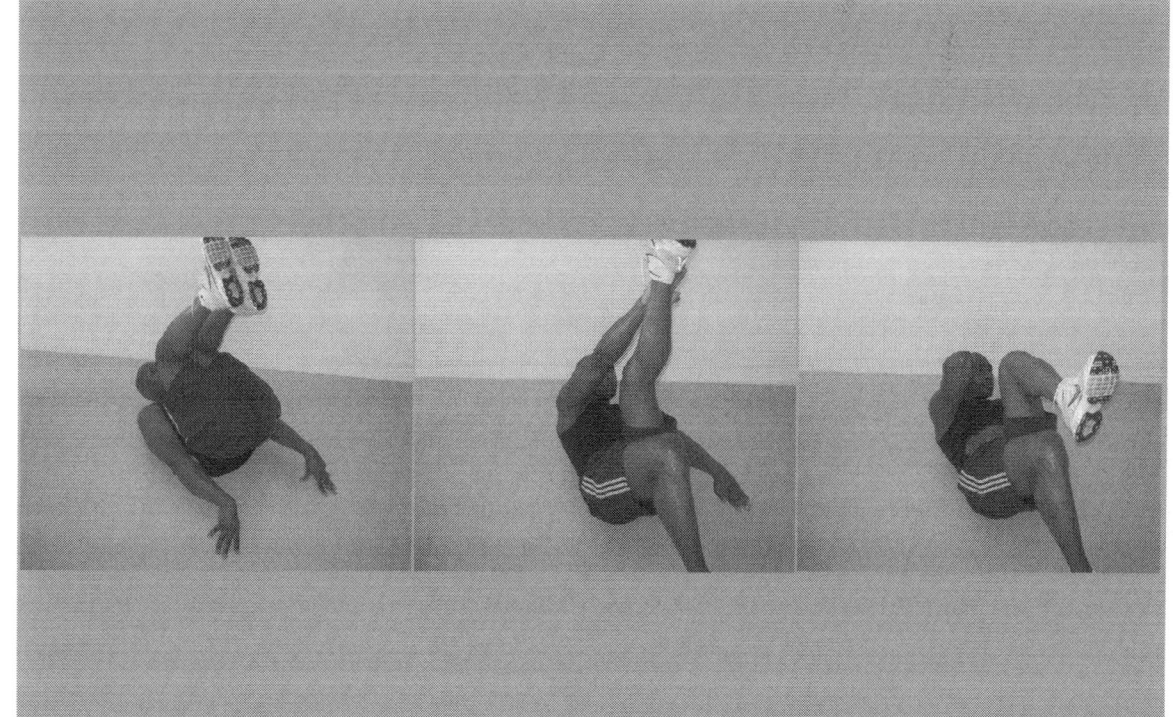

Hip Flexor Function

The hip flexors come into play on many ab exercises, such as reverse crunches. As you'll soon see, the hip flexors are important contributors, when you exercise the rectus abdominis. Upper and lower separation. Like I said, there's no real separation on upper and lower abs. Studies indicate that the upper rectus abdominis can work somewhat independently of the lower part of the muscle, as it does when you perform crunches. Or abdominal situps (feet extended not anchored) But when you work the lower portion, your upper rectus always comes into play, as in reverse crunches or across the body crunches.

Therefore, you should always work the lower area first, which brings both upper and lower sections into play. If you isolate the upper part first, you fatigue that area and make your lower-ab work much less effective—in much the same way that working forearms before biceps can limit your biceps efforts. For example, if you do crunches first and then reverse crunches, which works your upper rectus will be so fatigued from the crunches that it'll cause you to fail on the Reverse Crunches long before you fatigue your lower abs—it's one reason so many trainees lack lower-ab delineation:

They work lower abs last or do only crunches in their ab program. So here's just a few exercises that gets the job done. It works the muscles in union in order to get the best of both worlds.

Reverse Crunches

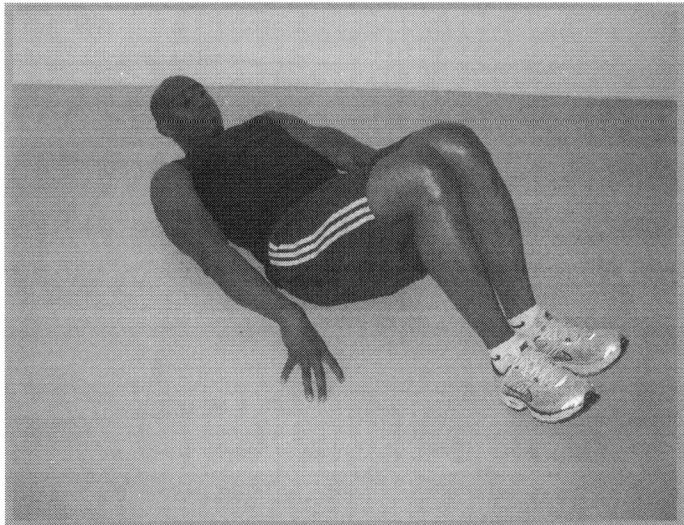

Start Position

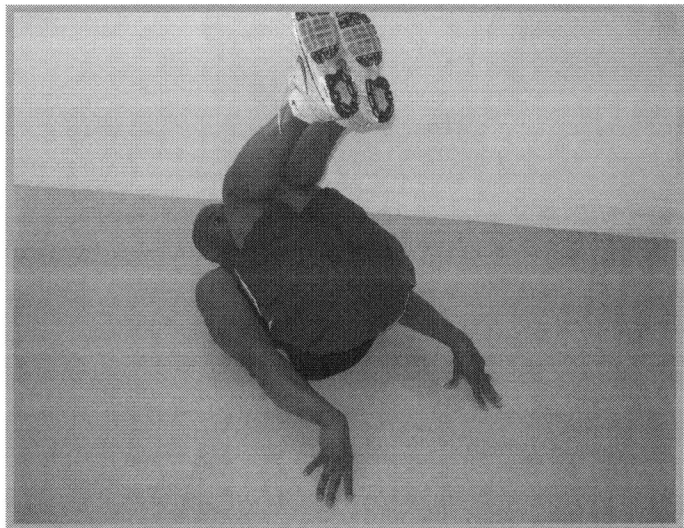

Finished Position

Start as shown in the start position picture. Then roll the hip as you bring the knees into the chest and continue for desired reps.

Across-The-Body Situps

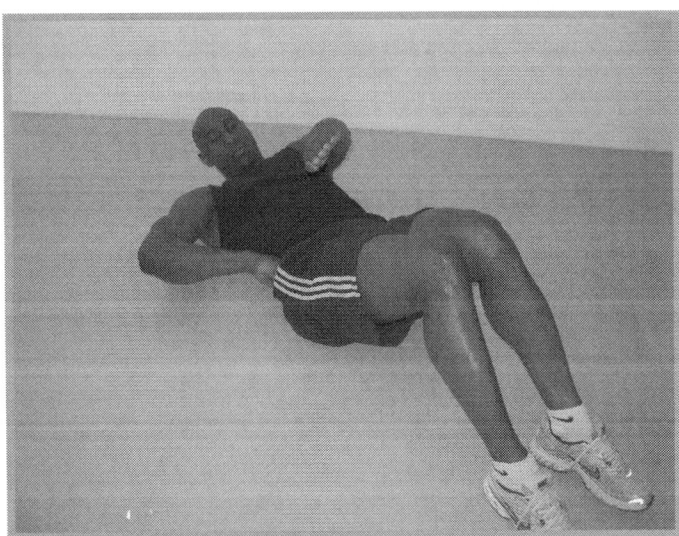

Start Position

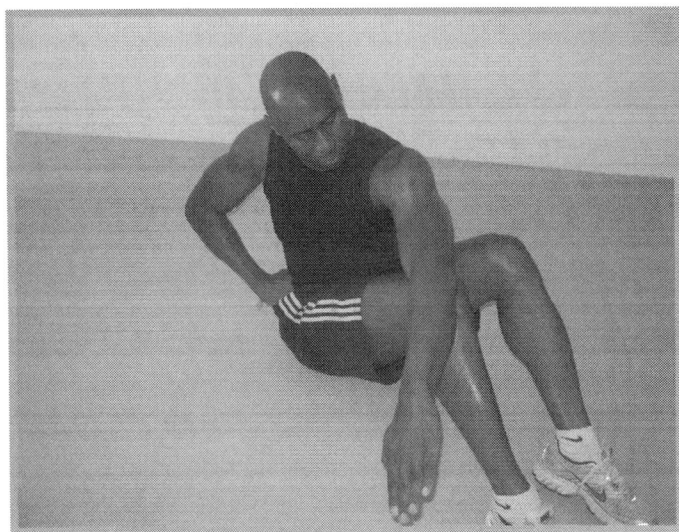

Finished Position

Start as shown in first picture. Now raise the upper body upwards and extend the left arm across the right knee as shown. This is a fine exercise for the entire abdominal wall as well as the obliques. After working one side for reps continue with the other in the same manner.

Across-The-Body Side Crunches

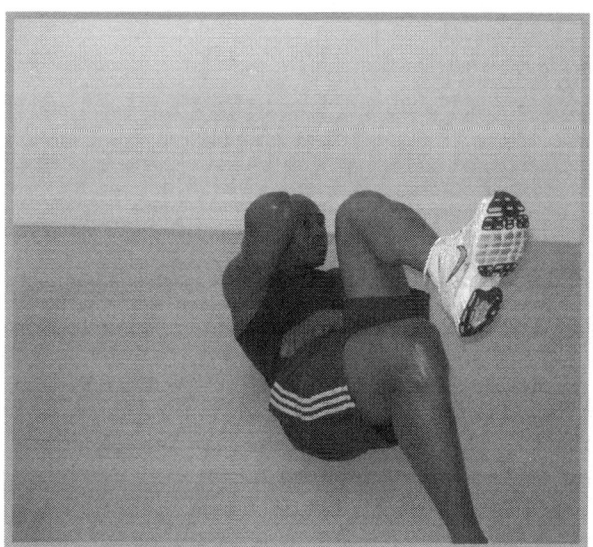

Start Position

Start off flat on the floor with right hand by the ear or behind the head, Knees together feet on floor, place the non-working arm on the floor or on the stomach. Now, rotate towards the left knee as shown while bringing it towards the elbow. While touching reverse the movement by going down and lowering the foot in line with the other leg. Perform for reps then change sides.

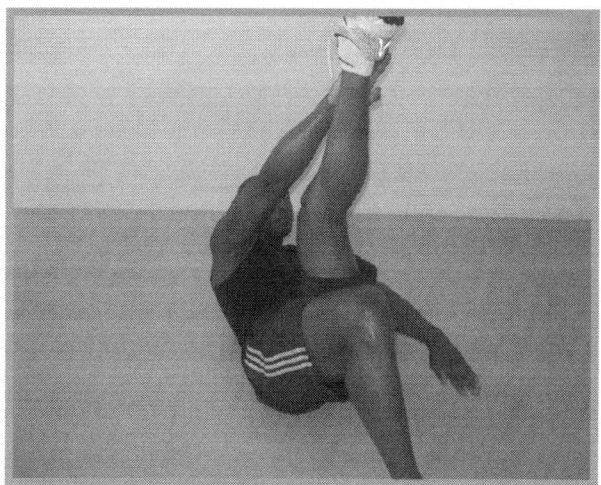

Another Version
Perform this version in the very same manner but extend the left leg upwards and extend the right hand upwards touching the ankle. Perform desired reps and change sides.

Stress Methods

Ten by Ten Method: Perform this stress method by performing ten complete full reps immediately followed by ten half reps from the start position to mid-point.

Double Impact Method: Perform this stress method by alternating one full rep immediately followed by a half rep. (one full and one half equals one rep)

Compound Isolation Method: Perform three sets of one exercise by itself. Then superset two other exercises. A superset is combining two movements back to back and then you rest.

Fiber Overload Training Method: Perform the exercise at the strongest muscle building signal, the Power Point. This means you are only training to the half point. Using the curl as an example, you curl from the starting position to the half way point, stop, and then push back down. Or with the push-up. You start at the bottom position you push half way up and then come back down again.

CHAPTER 4

Ten by Ten Method Phase One

Workout One: Monday, Wednesday and Friday
Workout Two: Tuesday, Thursday and Sunday

This First Plan is to be performed for 3 weeks. Ten by Ten Method. Perform 10 Full Reps followed by Ten Half Reps

Workout One PHASE ONE
Thigh Rows

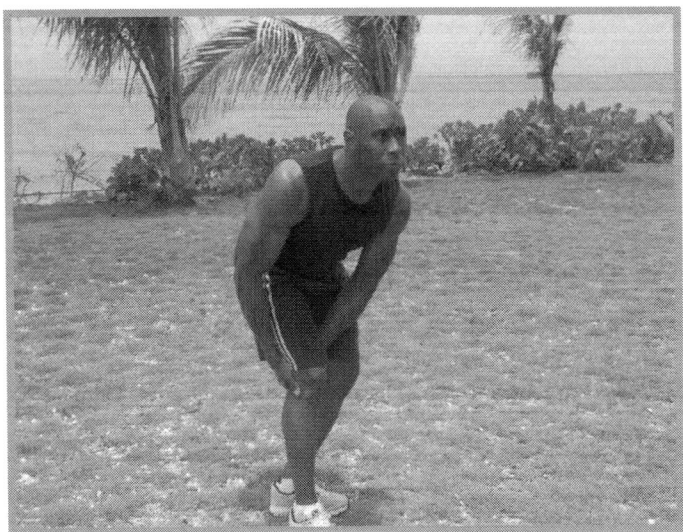

Start Position

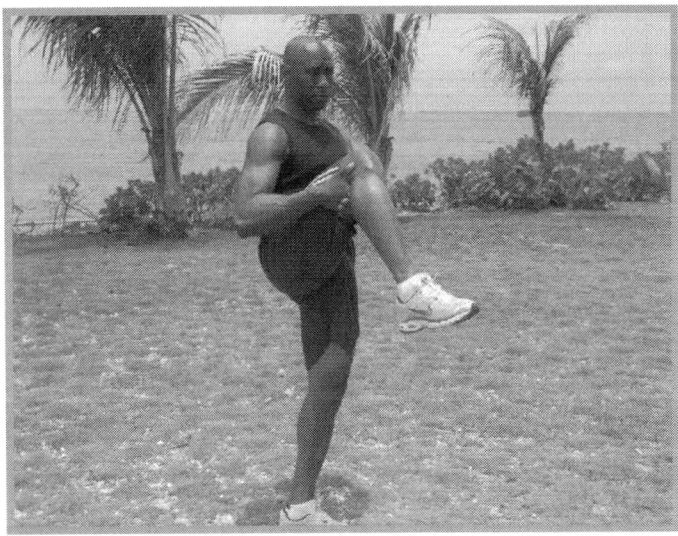

Finished Position
Full Reps Only 15-20 per leg

Three Chair Dips (Basic Upper Back)

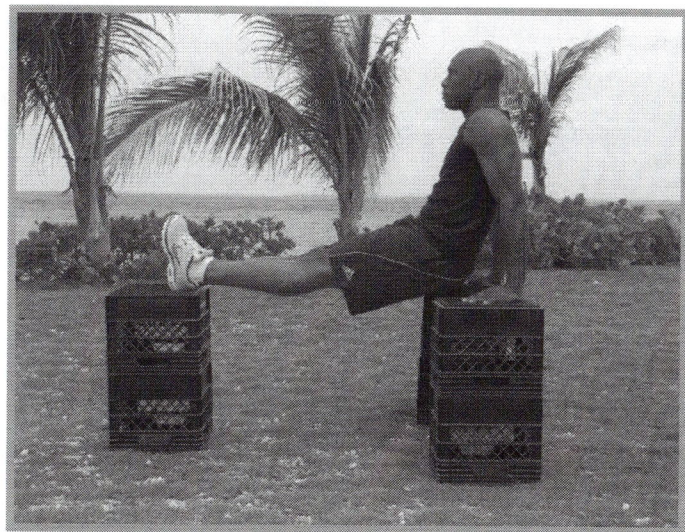

Start Position

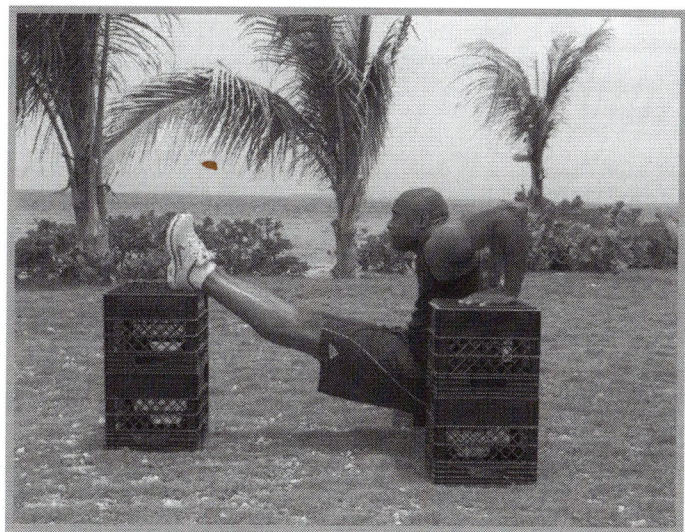

Finished Position

These are to be performed for full reps only. 3 Sets of 15 reps before moving to next exercise.

Stiff-Arm Pulldown (Isolation) Upper Back

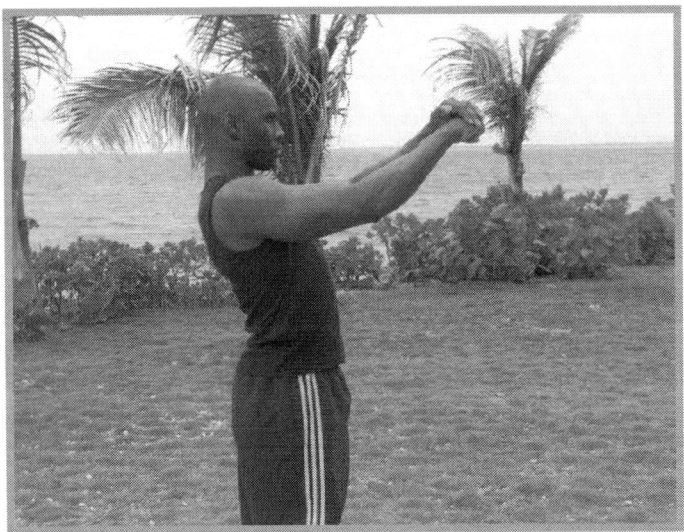

Start Position

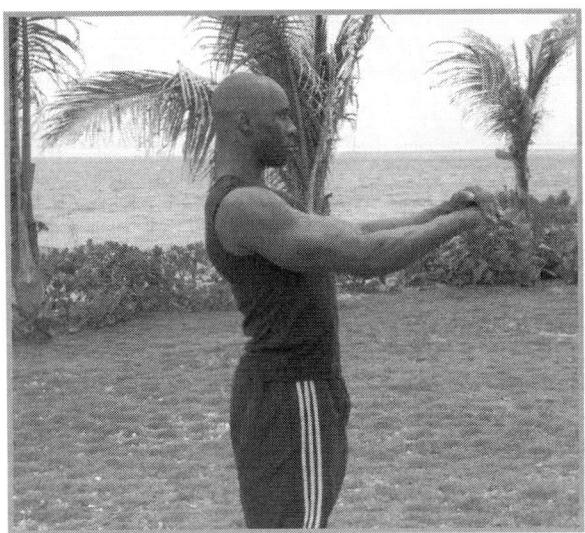

Mid-Point

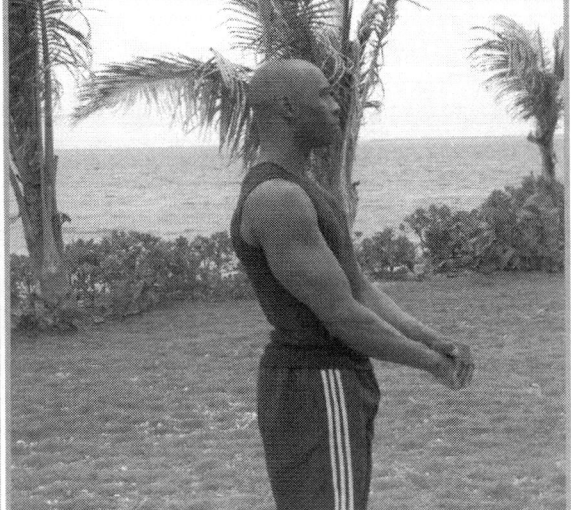

Finished Position

Perform 10 full reps, followed by 10 half reps from finished position to mid-point. Then switch hands and perform the 10 by 10 method again.

Across-The-Body Rows (Lats/Mid-Back)

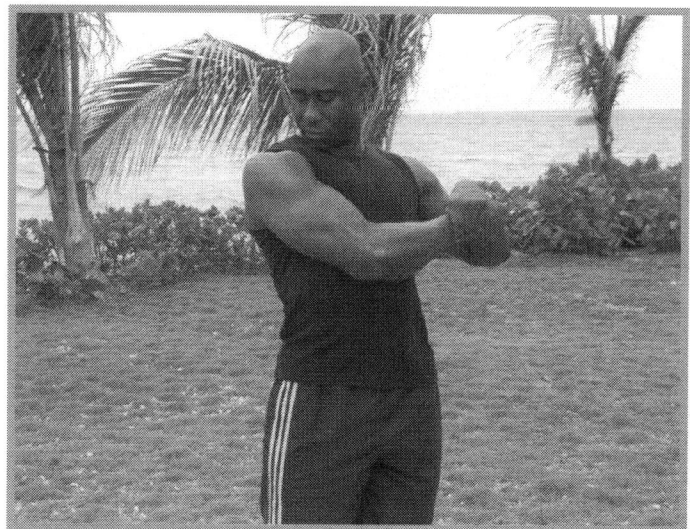

Start Position

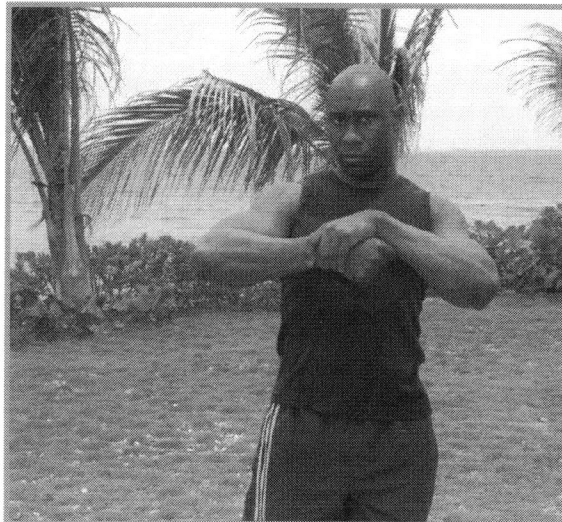

Mid-Point

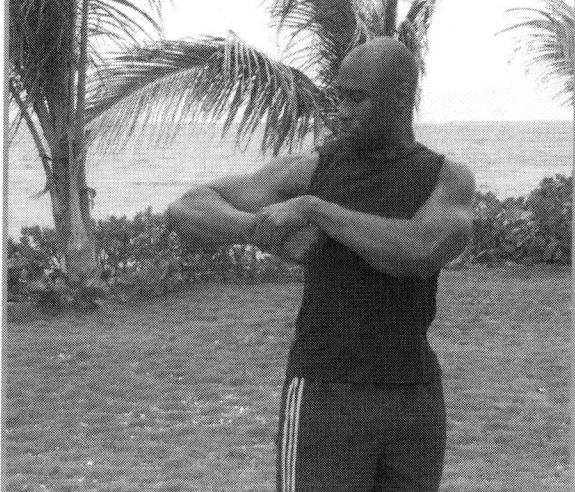

Finished Position

Perform 10 full reps, followed by 10 reps at the mid point to finished position. Then switch sides and repeat.

Decline Pushups (Basic/Stretch)

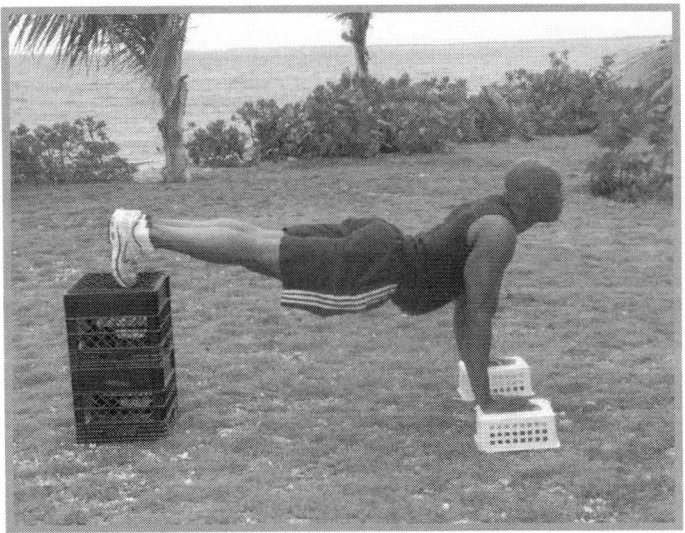

Start Position

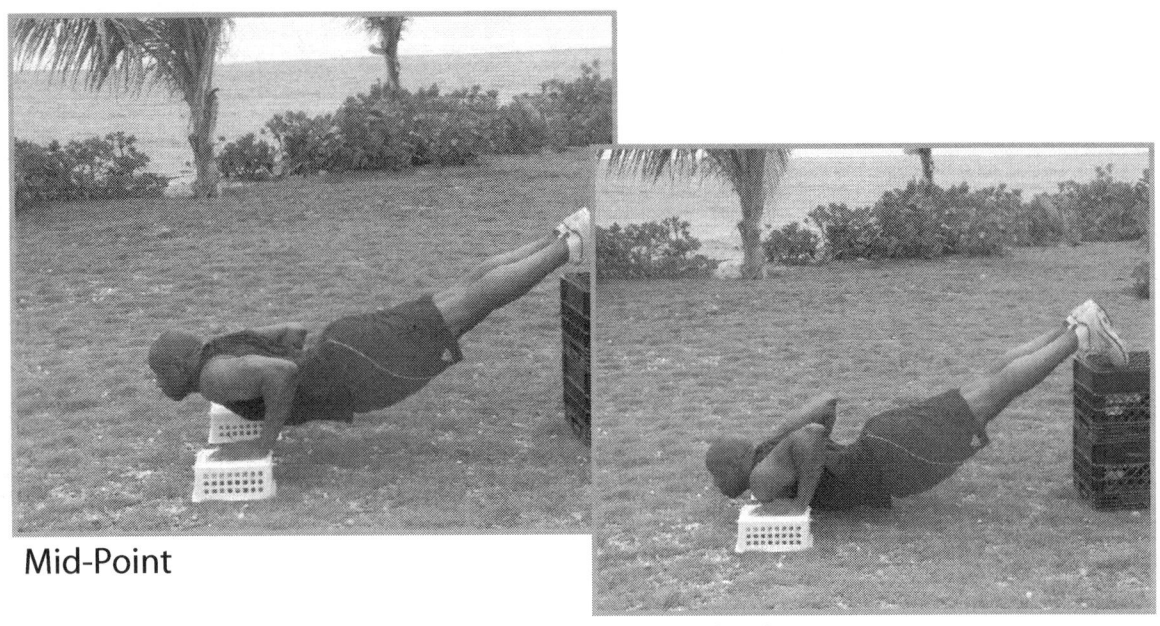

Mid-Point

Finished Position

Perform 10 full reps, followed by 10 half reps from the mid-point to finished position.

Liederman Press (Basic/Stretch/Isolation)

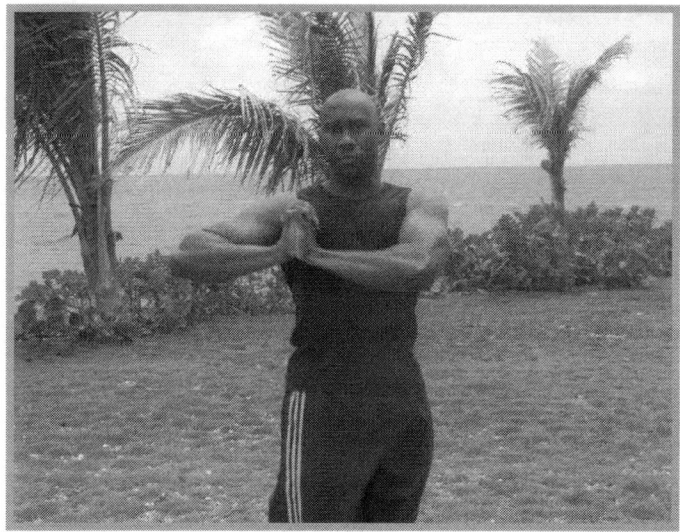

Start Position

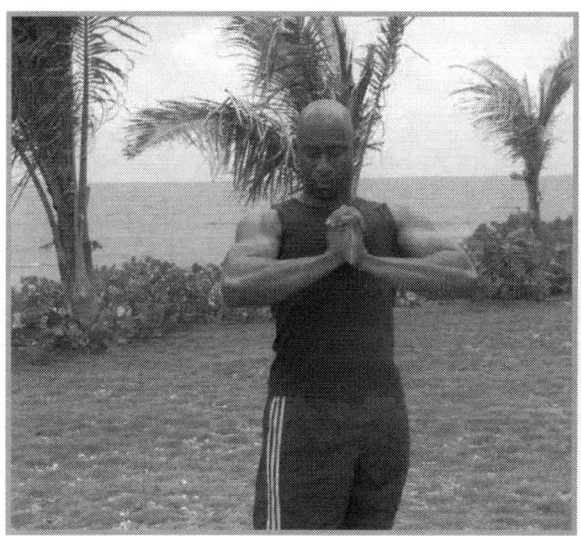

Mid-Point

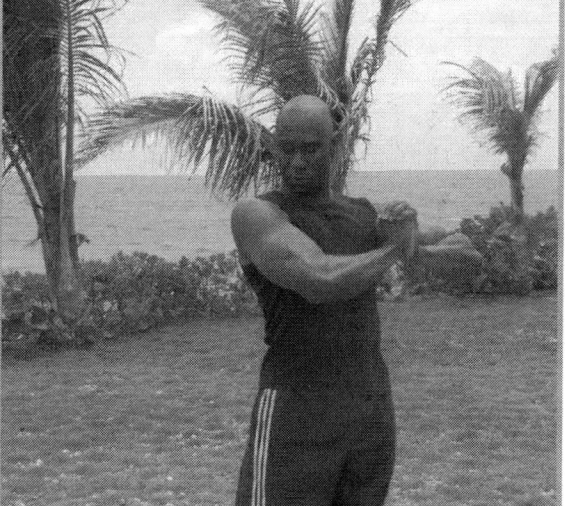

Finished Position

Perform 10 full reps from one shoulder to the next, then perform mini reps of 10 at the mid-point position, 2-3 inches within the middle chest.

Biceps (Basic)

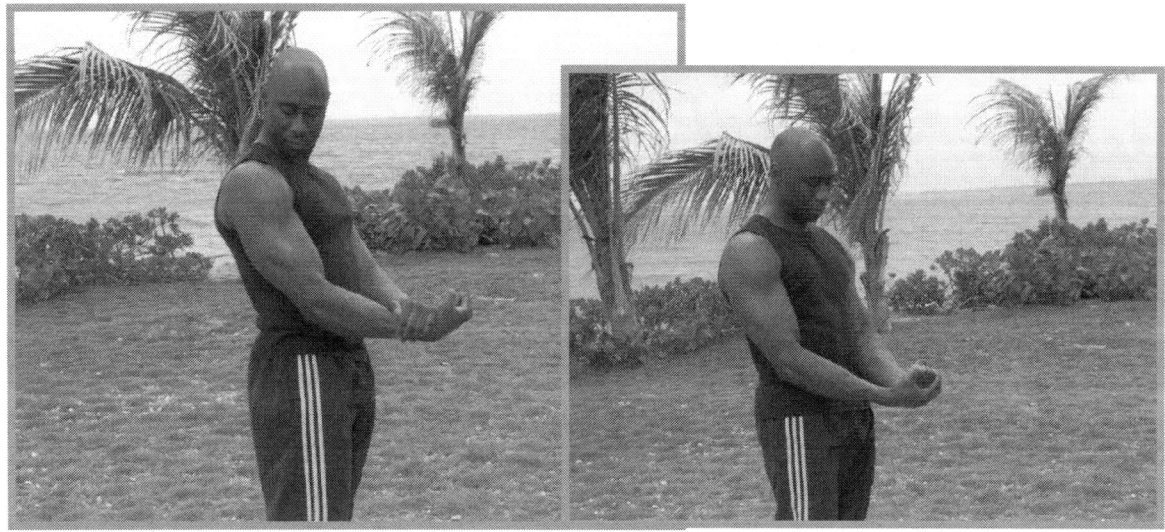

Start Position   Another Version

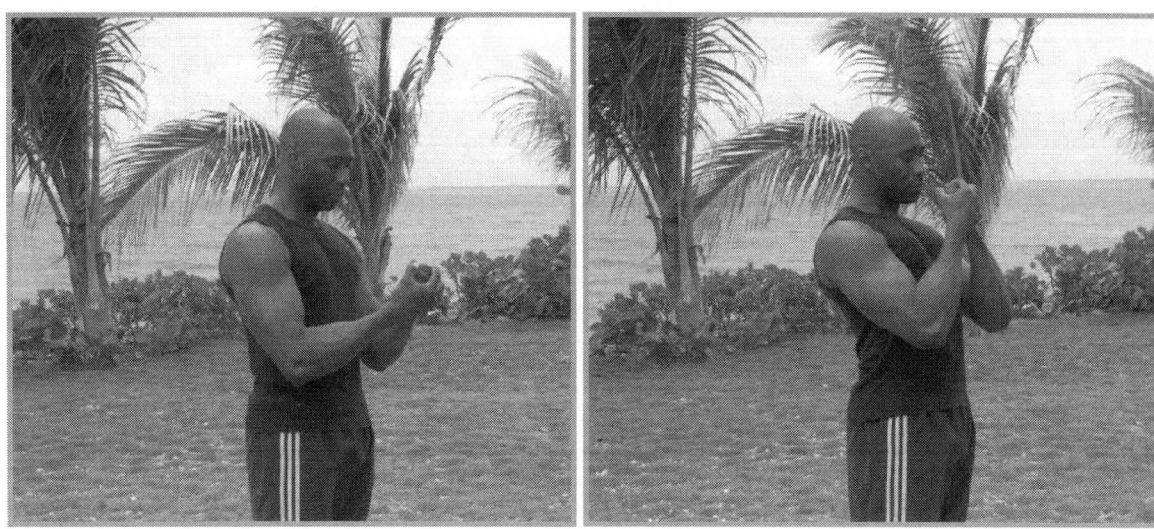

Mid- Point   Finished Position

Either holding onto the wrist or fist in palm as shown.. Perform 10 reps full range followed by 10 half reps. Bottom to mid point for another 10 reps. Continue with the other arm same format.

Reverse Curls (Forearms/Biceps Basic)

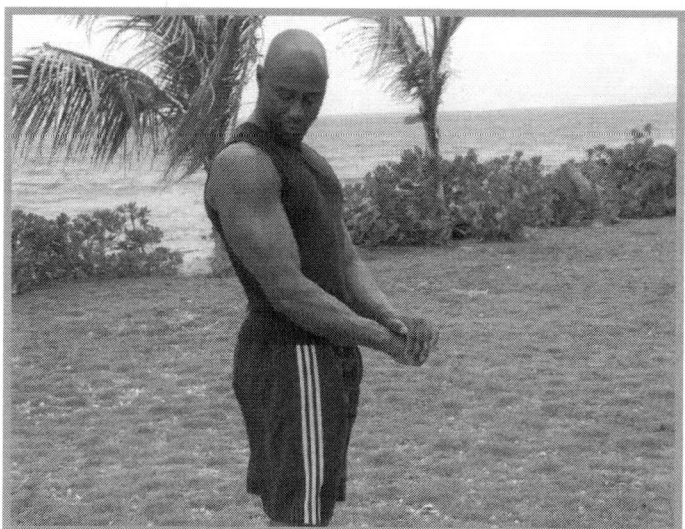

Start Position

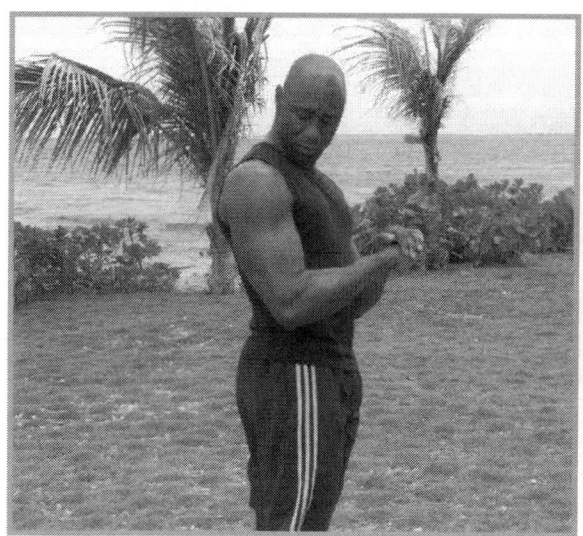

Mid-Point

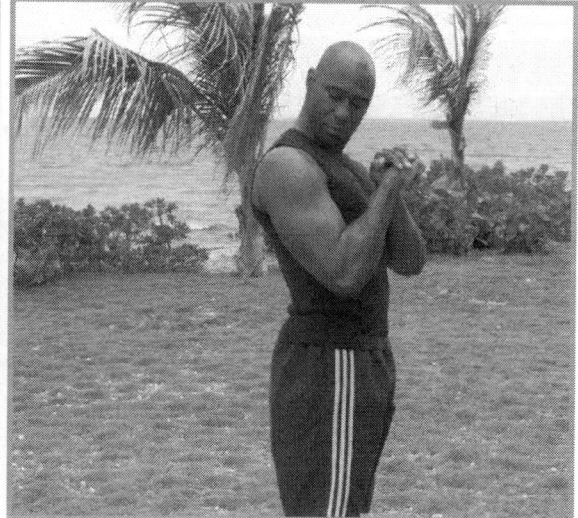

Finished Position

Perform 10 full reps followed by 10 half reps from the bottom position to mid point. The Bicep power point that promotes the strongest muscle-building signal. Then switch arms and repeat the 10 by 10 method.

Standing Calve Raises (Stretch/Contracted)

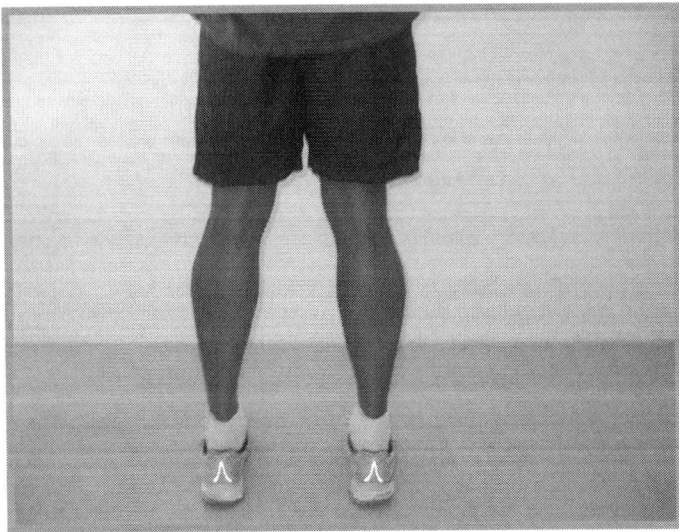

Start Position

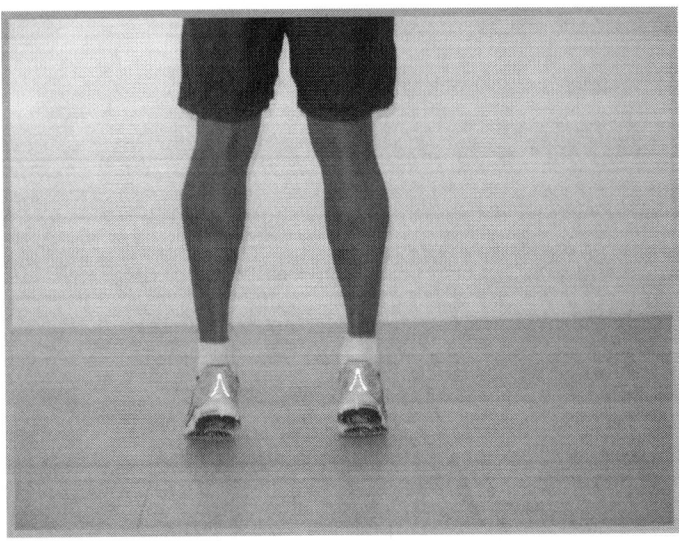

Finished Position

This exercise can be performed at the edge of your staircase. Perform 15 full reps followed by 15 top reps at the contracted finished position. By lowering the heels 2-3 inches from the top then driving it back up again. Great for increasing blood blockage and increasing tension on the working muscles.

Slanted Calf Raises

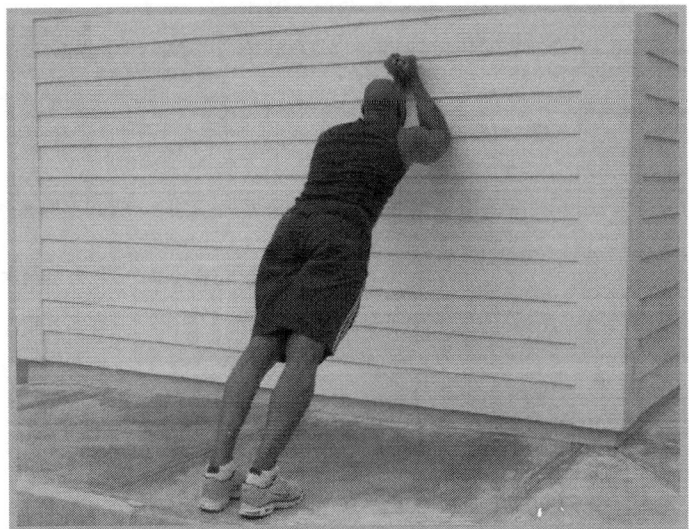

Start Position

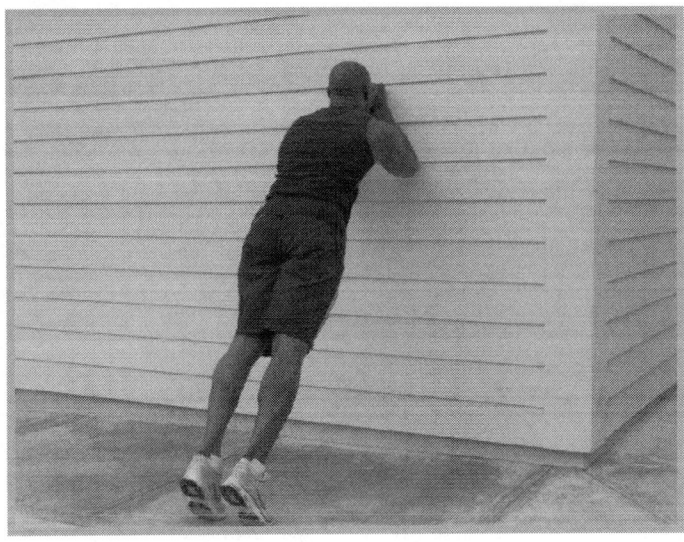

Finished Position

Perform this movement as before. Performing 15 full reps followed by 15 half reps at the top.

Workout Two

Ten by Ten Method Phase One

Workout Two   Tuesday Thursday Sunday

Shoulders (Isolation)

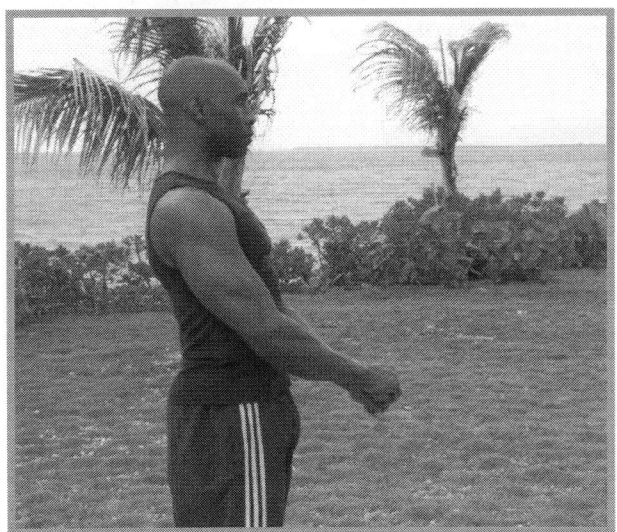
Start Position

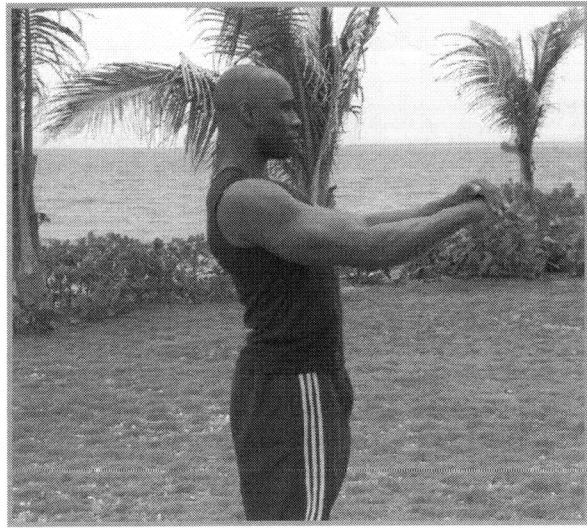
Mid-Point

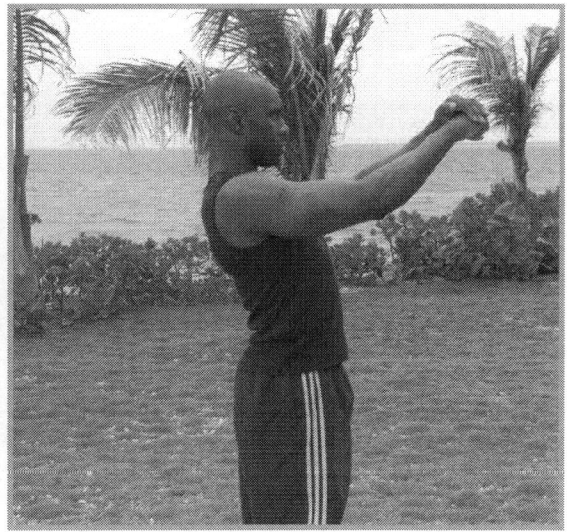
Finished Position

Perform 10 full reps followed by 10 half reps from the mid point to the finished position. Repeat on the other arm 10 by 10 method.

Rear Delts (Across-The-Body Pulls)

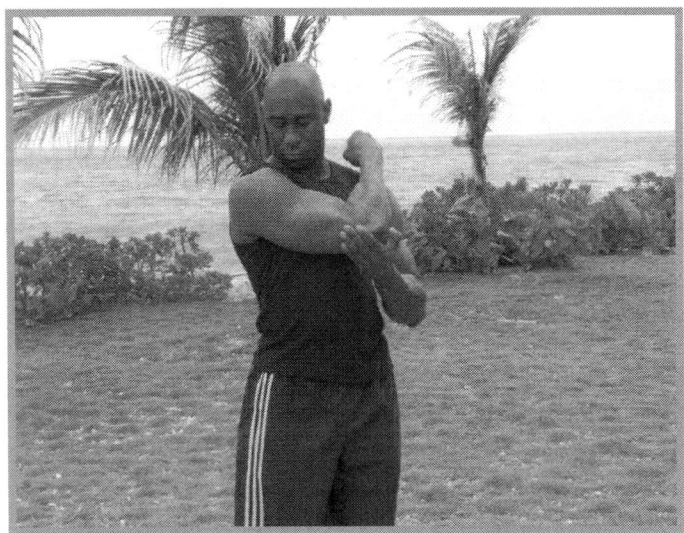

Start Position

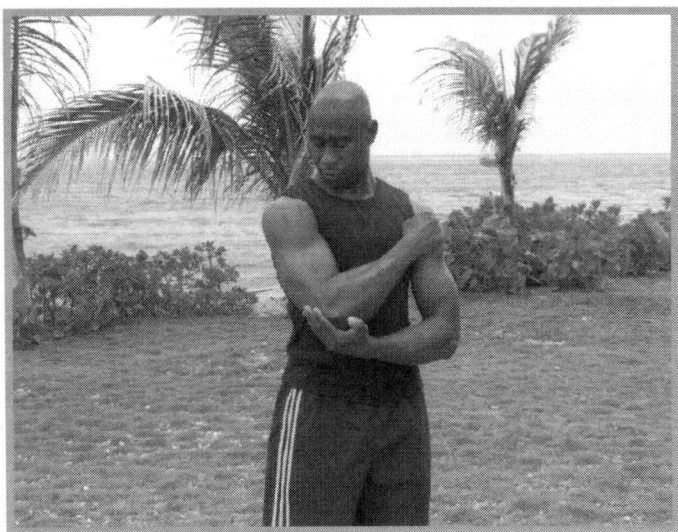

Finished Position

Full Reps Only. Sets of 10-15 reps per side.

Shoulders (contracted)

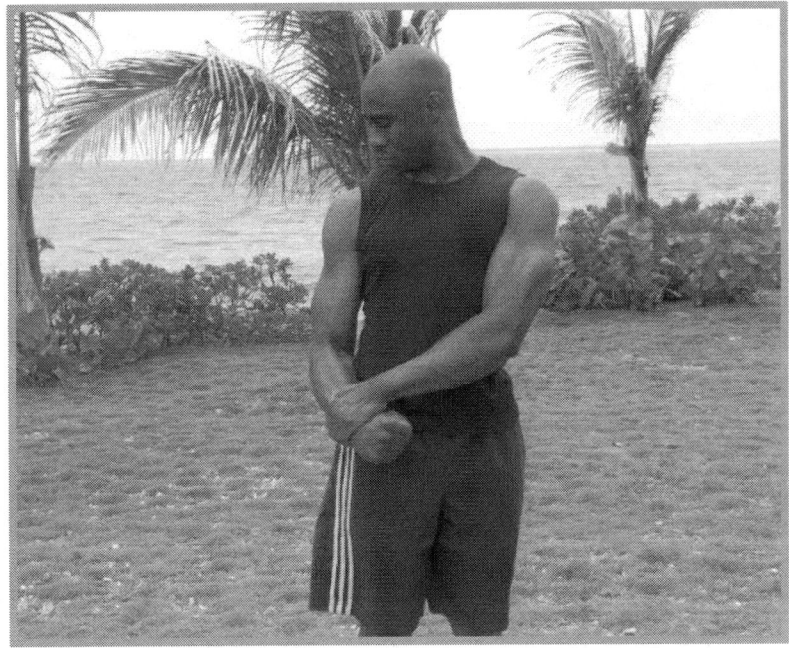

Start Position

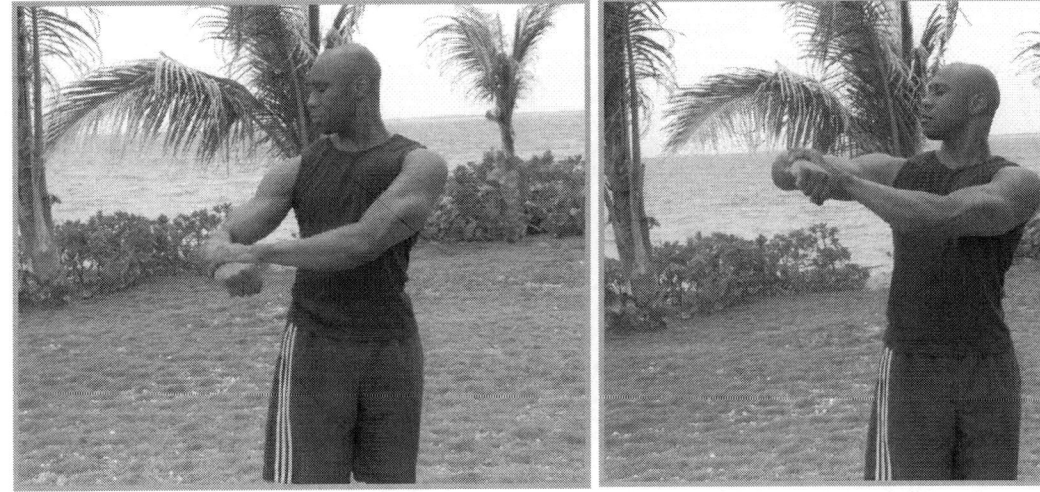

Mid-Point   Finished Position

Perform 10 full reps followed by 10 reps from mid point to finish position. After working one side work the other shoulder for another 10 by 10.

Neck Forward Press (Upper Traps)

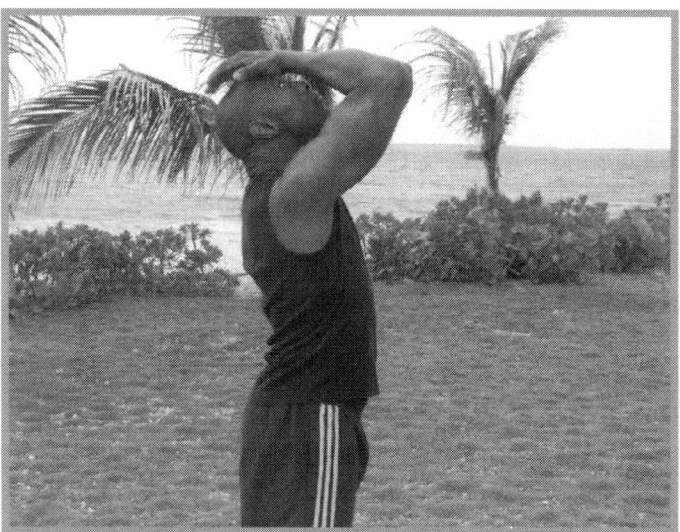

Start Position

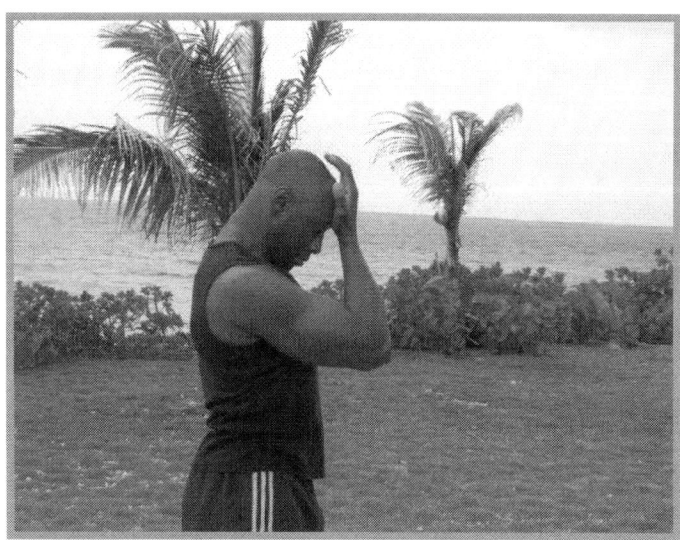

Finished Position

Start the exercise as shown but perform full reps only in one direction. 15-20 reps

Neck Rear Press (Upper Traps)

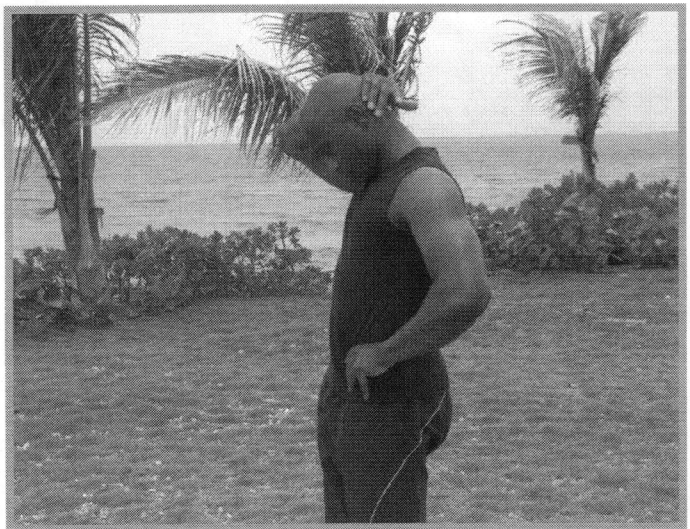

Start Position

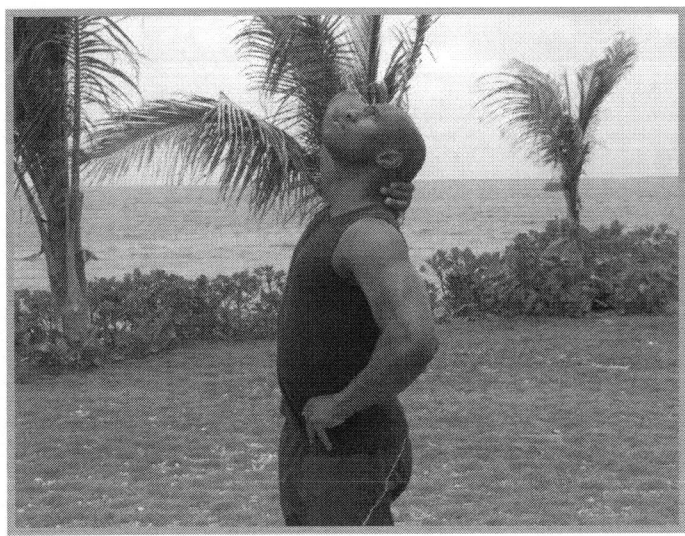

Finished Position

Perform full reps only. 15-20 reps are best!

Triceps Forward Extension (Basic) Lateral Head

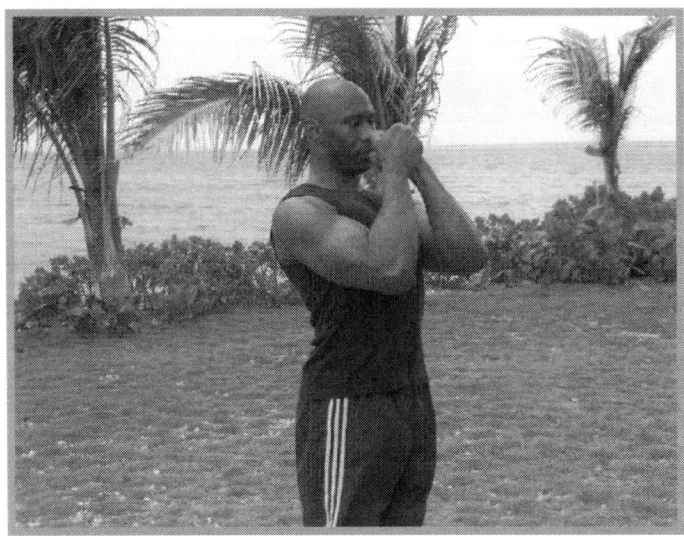

Start Position

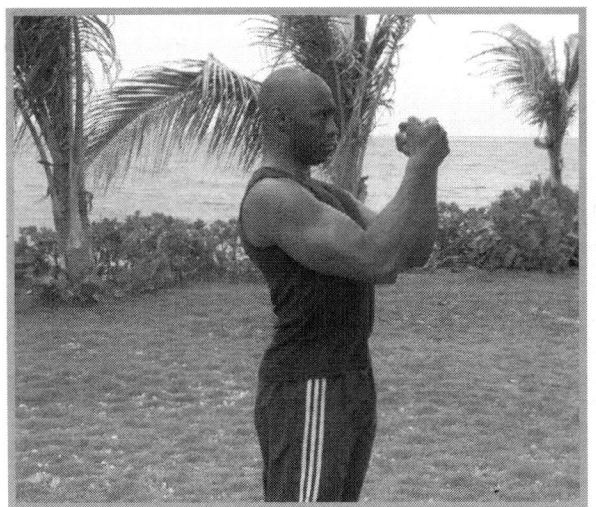

Mid-Point

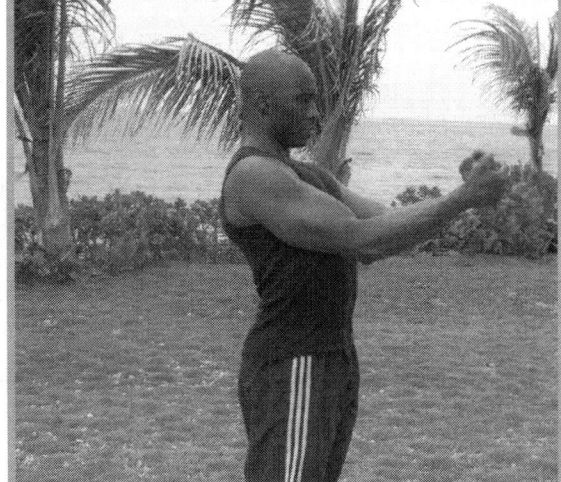

Finished Position

Perform 10 full reps, followed by 10 reps from the mid point to finished position. Then switch arms and perform the same format.

Triceps (Isolation) Tricep Pressdown (long/medial head)

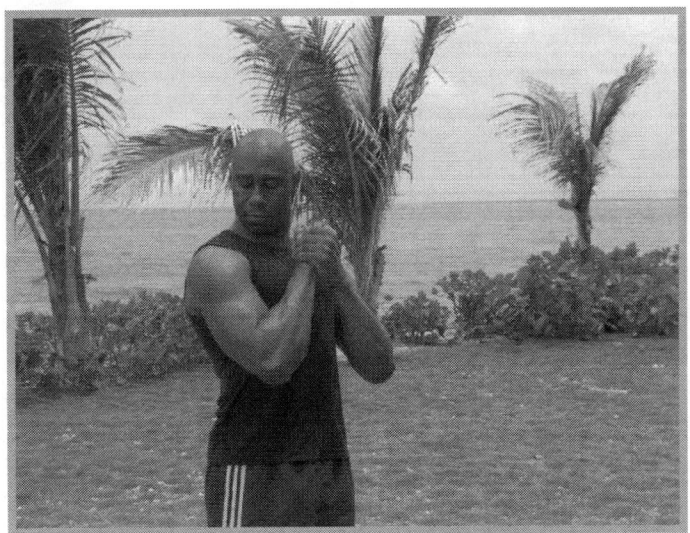

Start Position

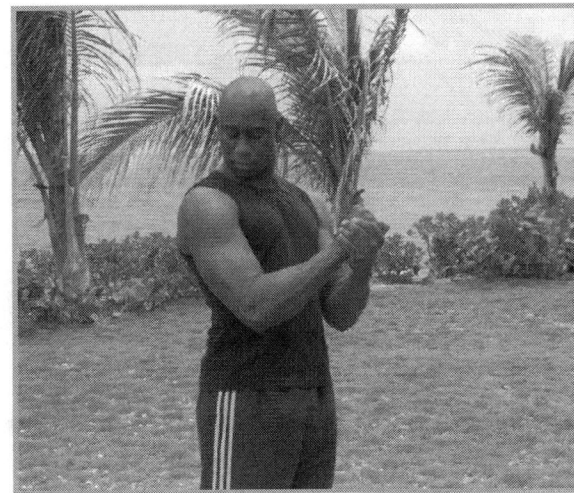

Mid-Point

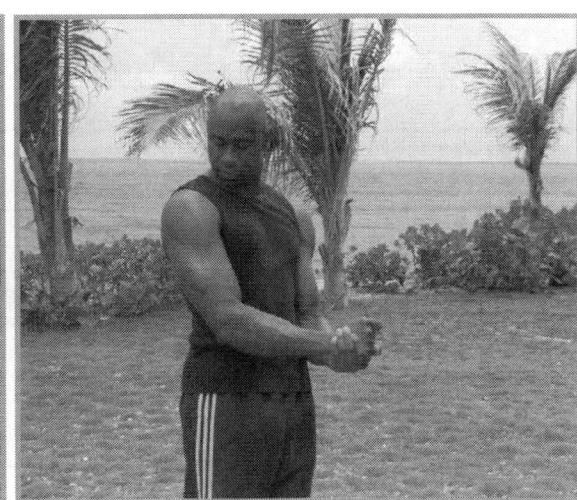

Finished Position

Perform 10 full reps followed by 10 reps from the mid point to finished position. After desired reps switch arms and repeat the same format.

Triceps Over-Head Press (Stretch) (long/medial head)

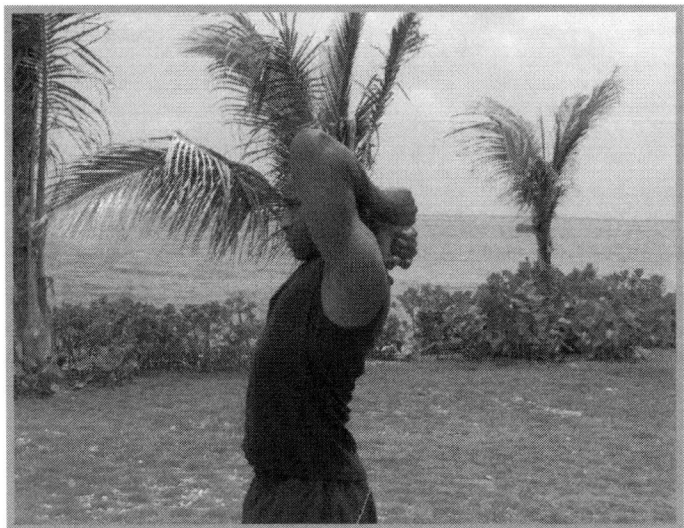
Start Position

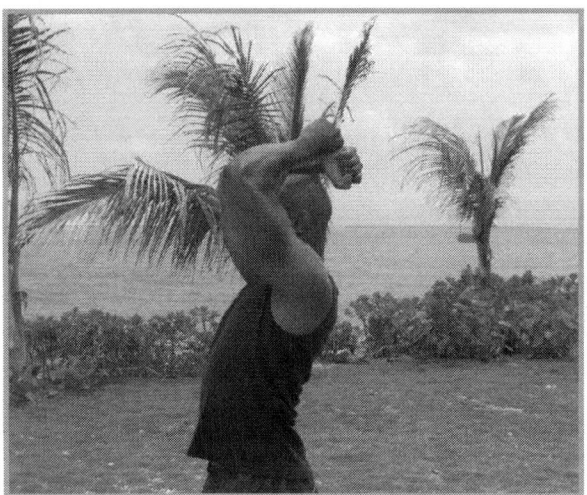
Mid-Point

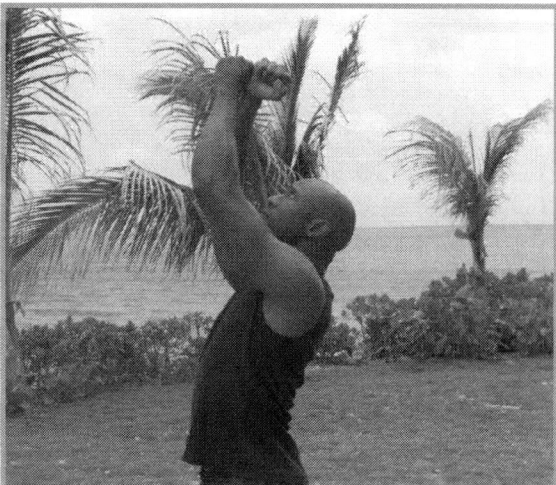
Finished Position

Perform 10 full reps followed by 10 reps from the start position to finished position resisting in both directions. Switch arms and continue same format. This exercise place undue stress on the tendons due to the position so caution should be used on tension. Hard (Heavy) Tension isn't needed! Please avoid at all cost! If not tendonitis will be the result.

Thighs   Regular Squats (Basic)

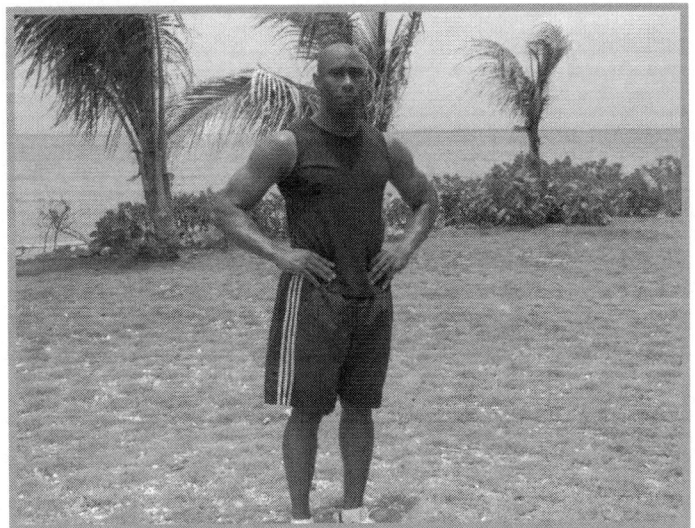

Start Position

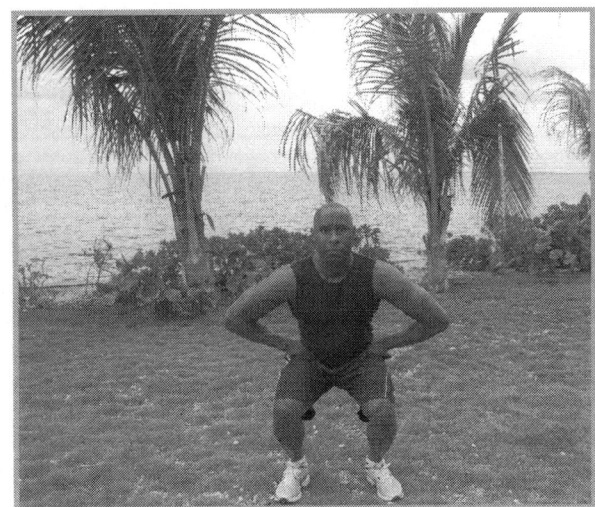

Mid-Point

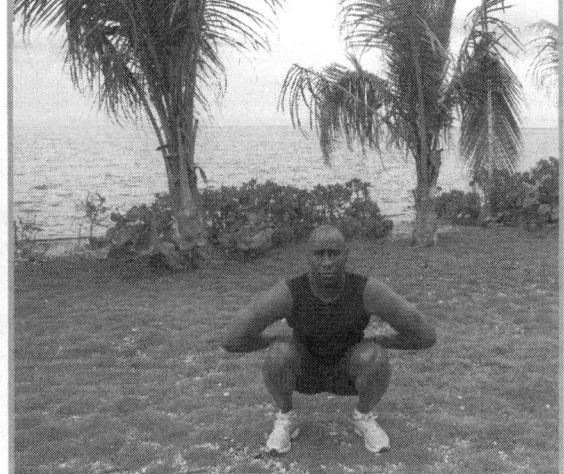

Finished Position

Perform 10 full reps followed by another 10 reps from mid point to finish position. (No Bouncing)

Resisted leg Extensions (Contracted)

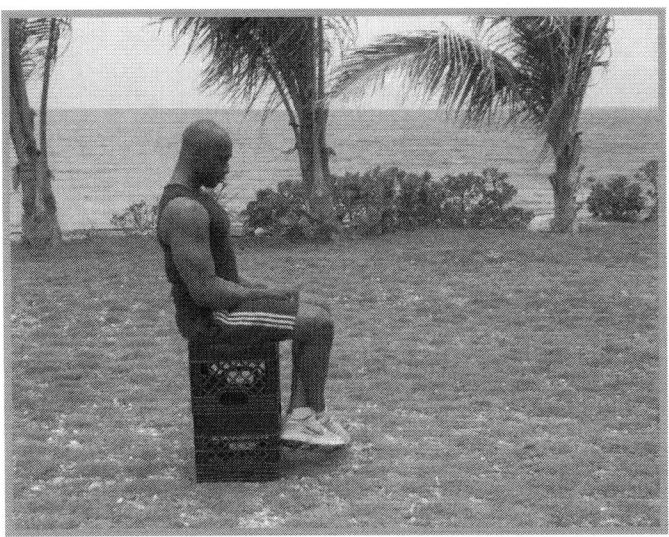

Start Position

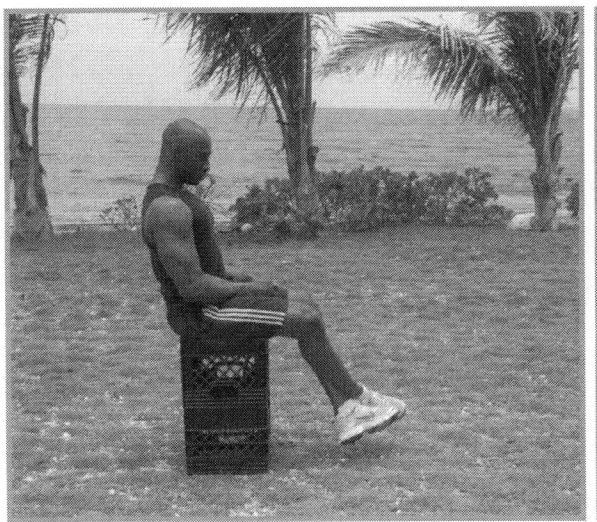

Mid-Point

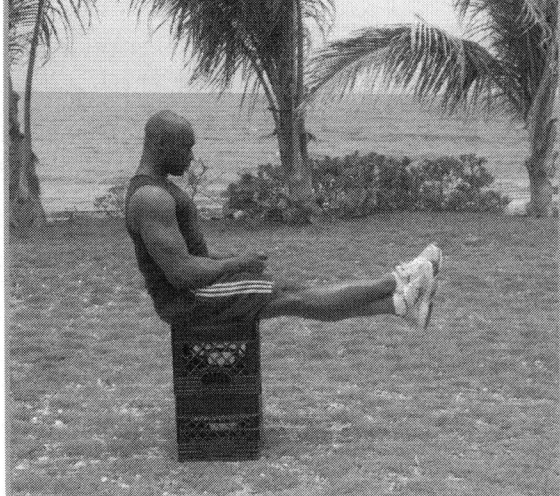

Finished Position

Perform 10 full reps followed by 10 reps from mid point to finished position. Switch legs and repeat in the same format. Maintain Tension and force on the up phase only.

Hamstrings (Isolation)

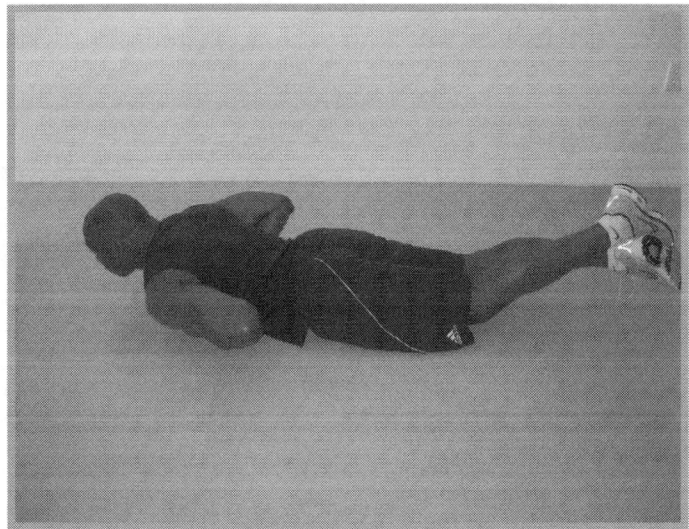

Start Position

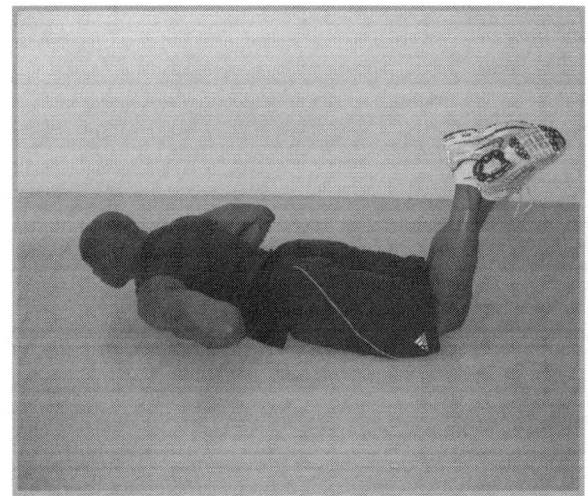

Mid-Point

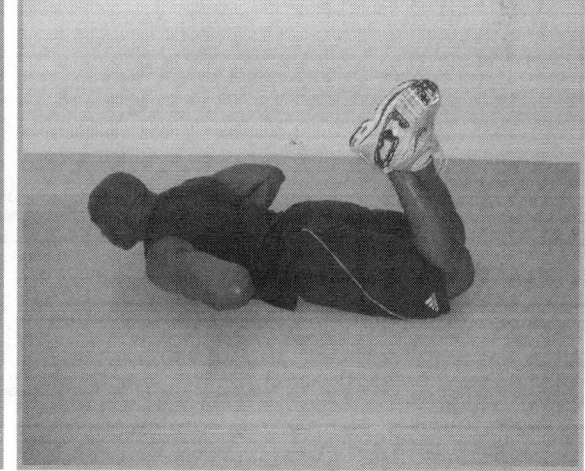

Finished Position

Perform 10 full reps followed by 10 reps from the mid point to finished position. Resist in one direction only.

Calves Slanted Calve Raises (Stretch)

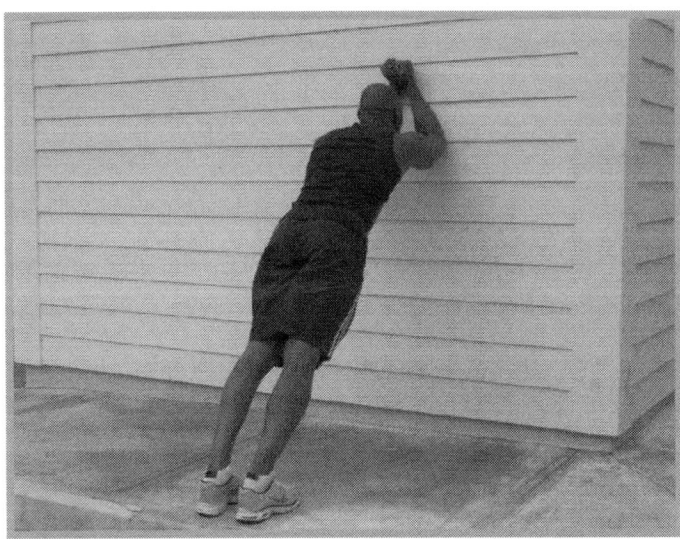

Start Position

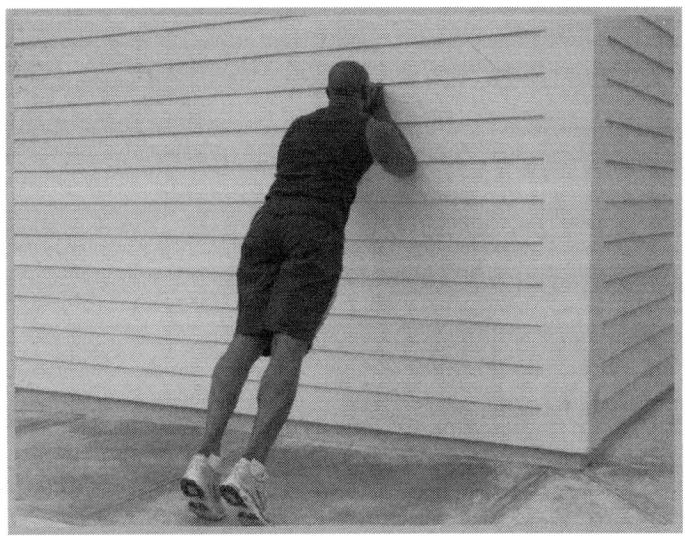

Finished Position

Perform 15 full reps, Then raise to the fully contracted position lower 2 inches and press back up again working in that position for 20 mini reps.

Chapter 5
Double Impact Method Powerpoint Training Phase Two

Workout One   Monday Wednesday and Friday
Workout Two   Tuesday Thursday Sunday
Perform this Phase for 3 weeks

Workout One Phase Two

Decline Press (Basic)

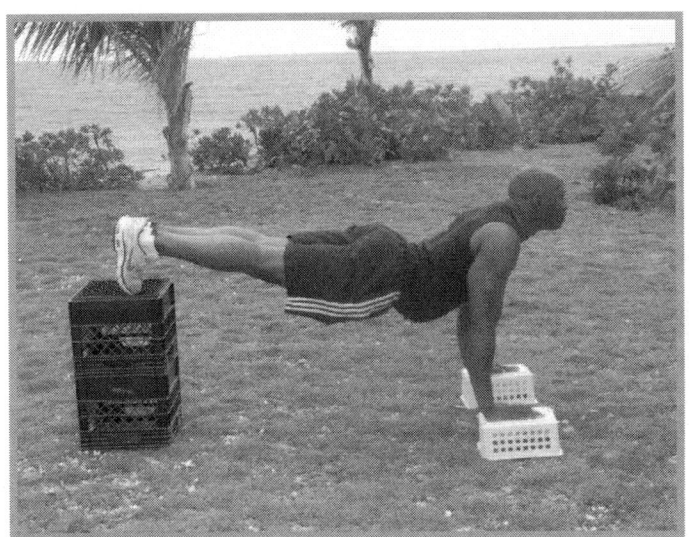

Start Position

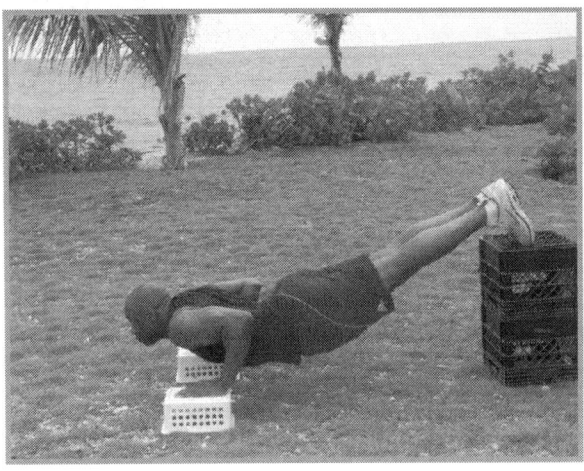

Mid-Point

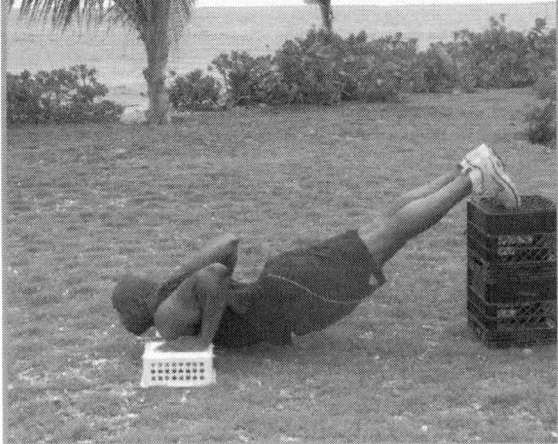

Finished Position

Double Impact Method: Start your reps for this exercise at the bottom position to mid point lower then press all the way up to start position. That's one rep. Perform 10 reps total 3 sets

Upper Chest (Stretch/Contracted)

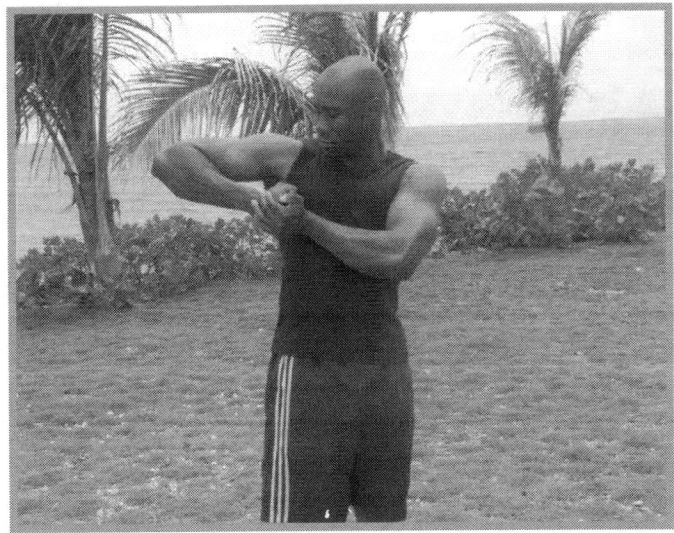

Start Position

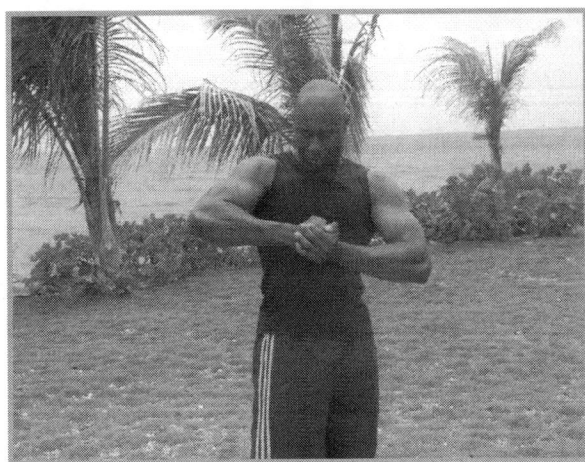

Mid-Point

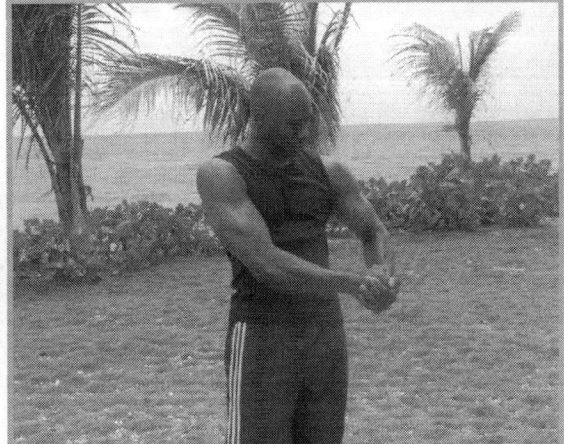

Finished Position

Perform full reps only. Resist in both directions before switching arms. 12 reps each side 2 sets

Shoulders (Basic)

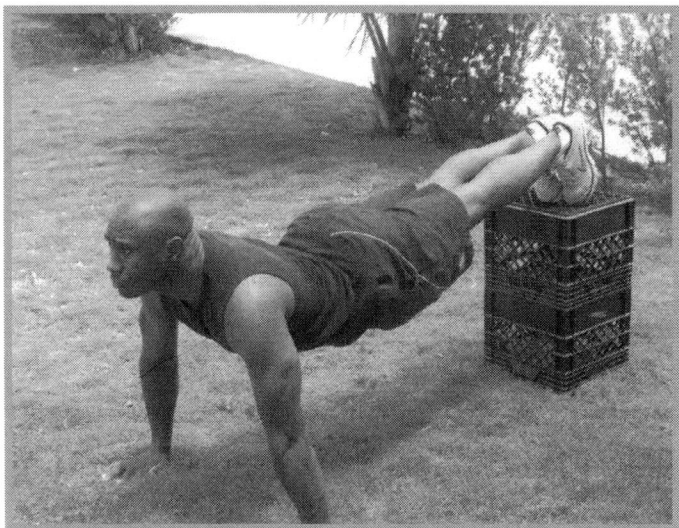

Start Position

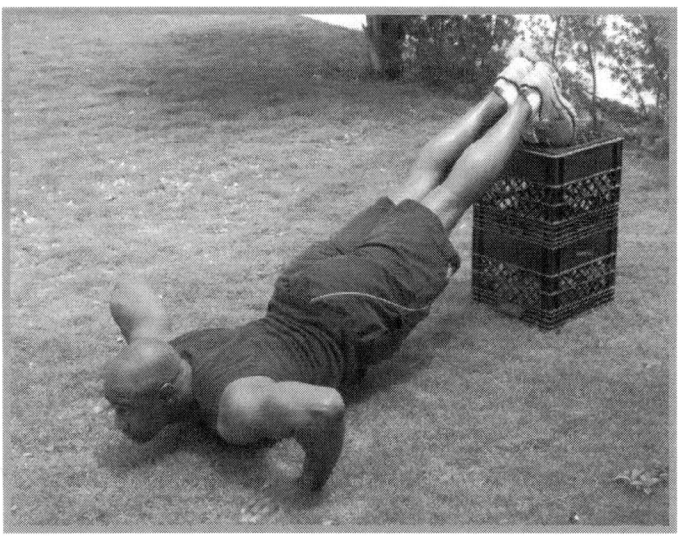

Finished Position (Mid-Point not shown)

Double Impact Method: Start this movement at the finished position pressing half way up, lower and perform a full rep. Remember one half rep followed by one full rep equals one rep. Perform 12 reps total 3 sets

Resisted Stiff Arm Pulldown (Contracted)

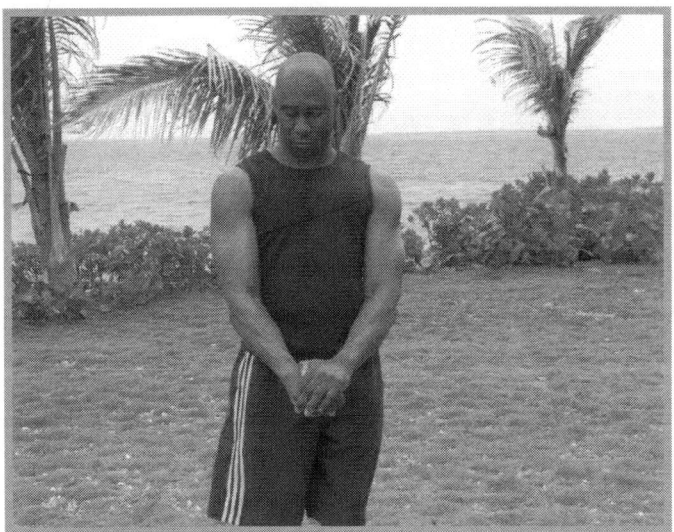

Start Position

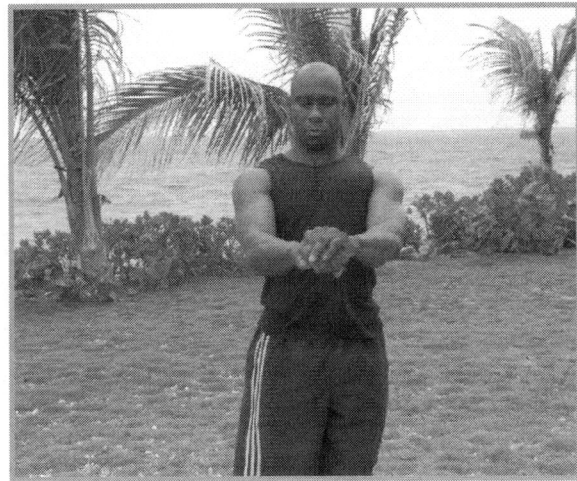

Mid-Point

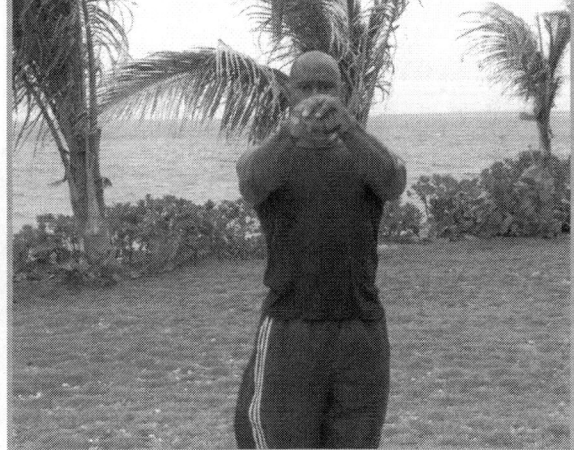

Finished Position

Double Impact Method: Start your reps for this exercise at the bottom position to mid point lower then press all the way up to start position. That's one rep. Perform 12 reps total 3 sets

Resisted Lateral Raises (Contracted)

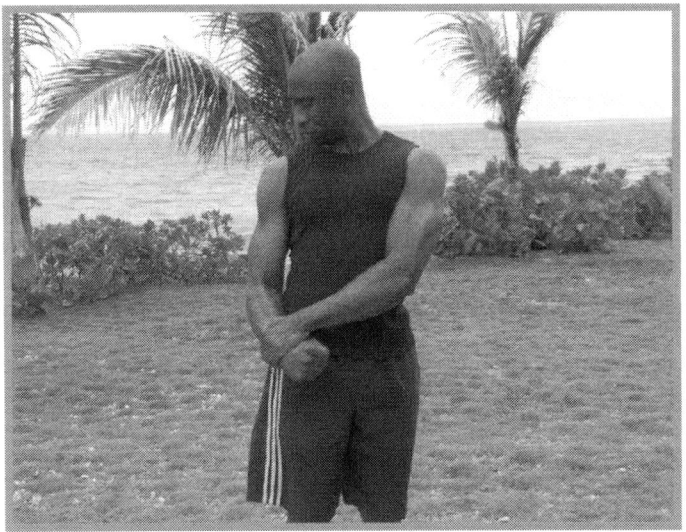

Start Position

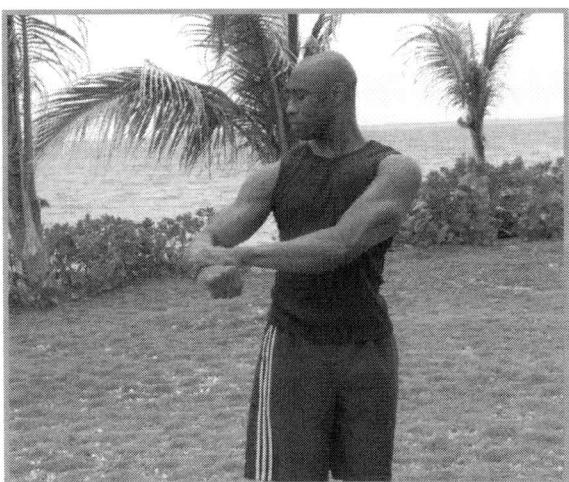

Mid-Point

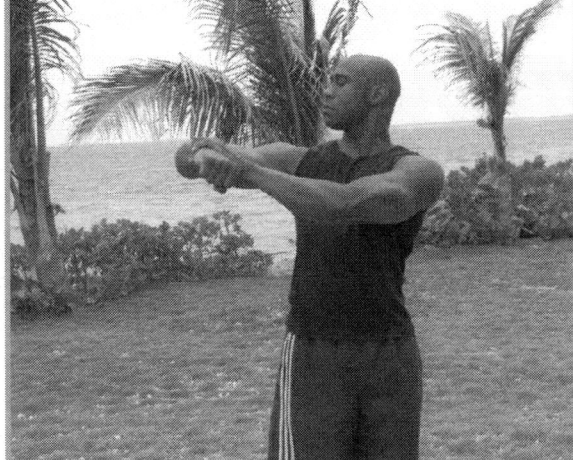

Finished Position

Double Impact Method: Raise the arm upward towards the finished position lower to mid point and drive it up again to the finish position lower and repeat. 12 reps total 2 sets

Across-The-Body Rows (Rear delts/Mid-Back, Lats)

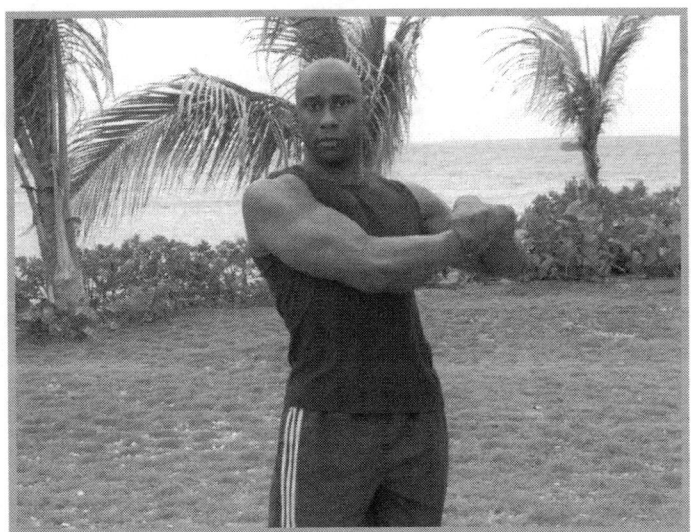

Start Position

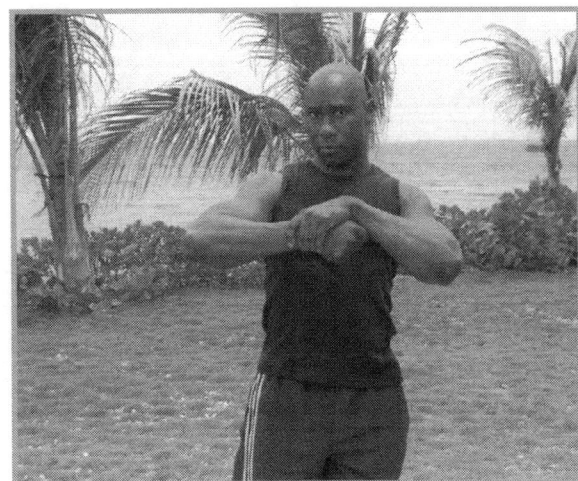

Mid-Position

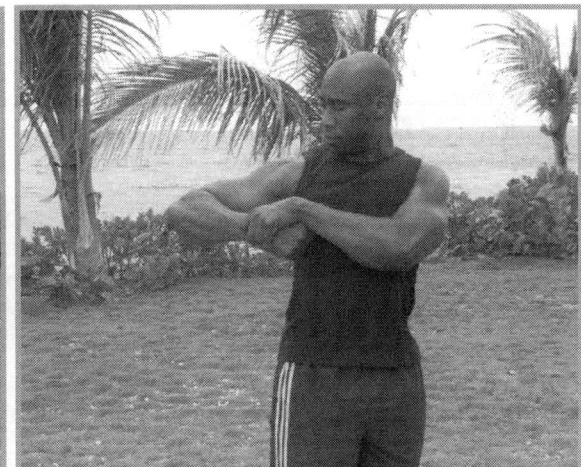

Finished Position

Perform full reps only 15 reps each side. 3 sets

Resisted Reverse Curls Basic (Forearms/Biceps)

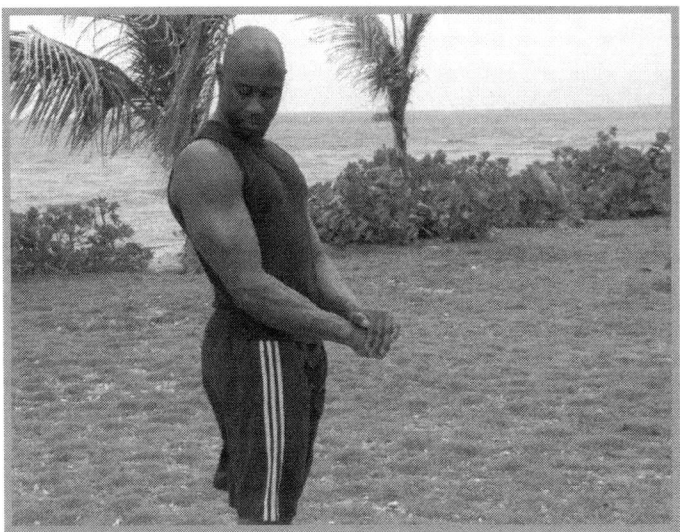

Start Position

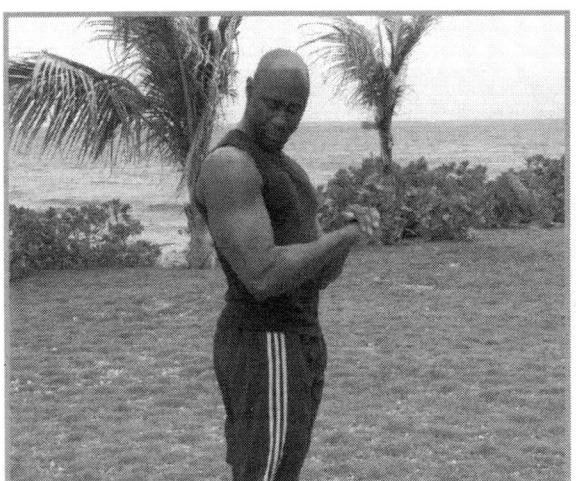

Mid-Point

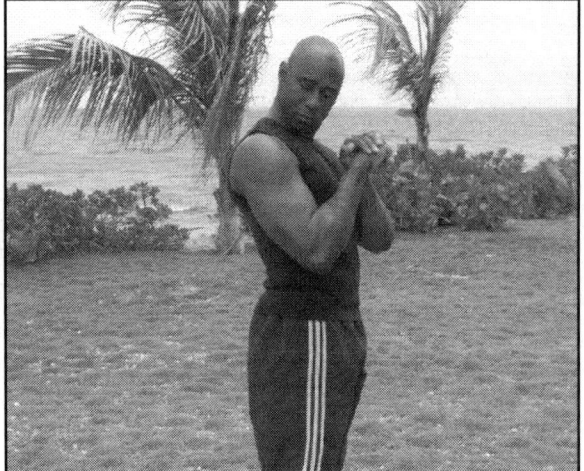

Finished Position

Double Impact Method: Start your reps for this exercise at the bottom position to mid point lower then curl all the way up to start position. That's one rep. Perform 12 reps total 3 sets each

Resisted Palm Up Curl (Basic)

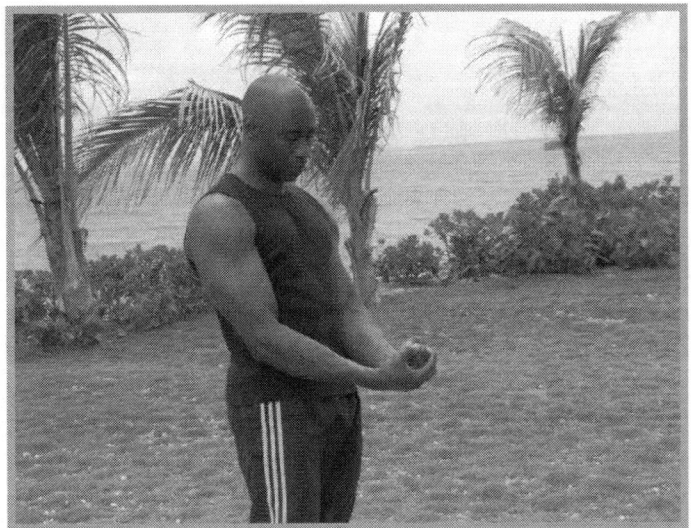

Start Position

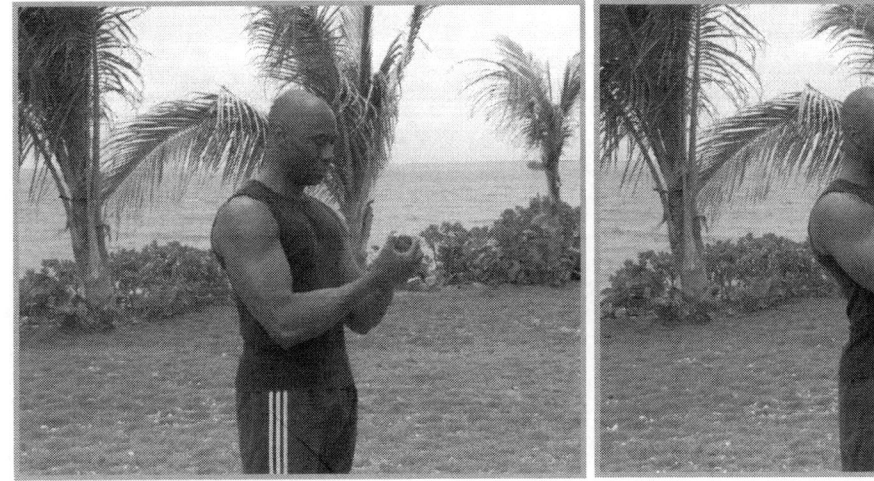

Mid-Point   Finished Position

Double Impact Method: Start your reps for this exercise at the bottom position to mid point lower then curl all the way up to start position. That's one rep. Perform 12 reps total 2 sets

Resisted Concentration Curls (Contracted)

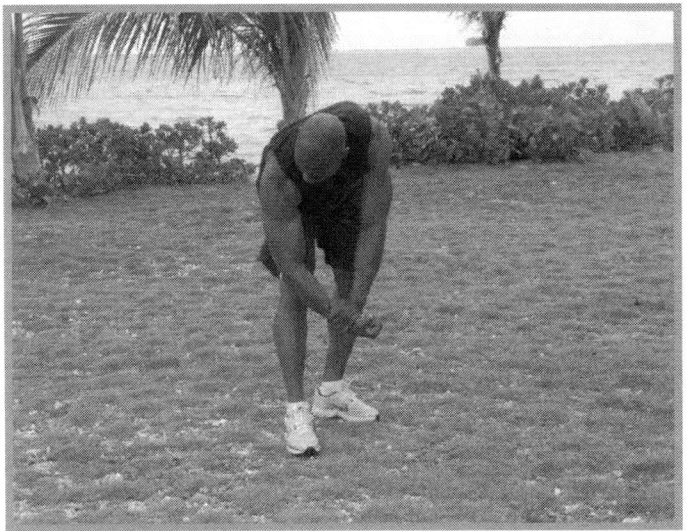

Start Position

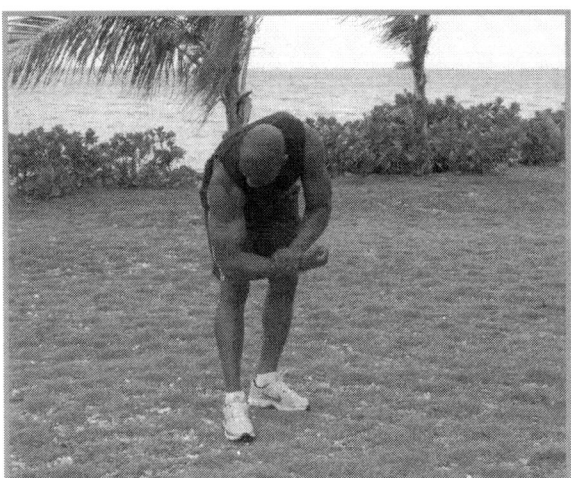

Mid-Point

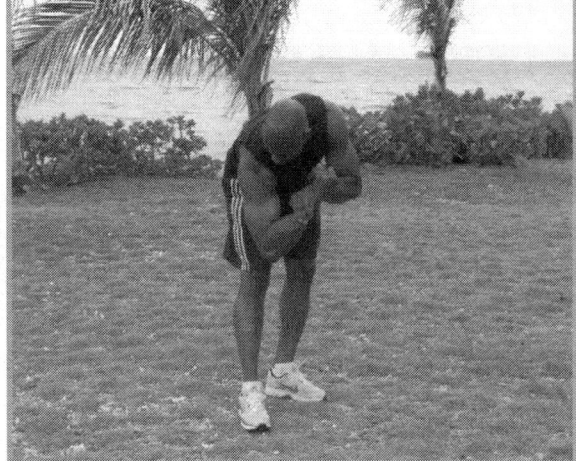

Finished Position

Double Impact Method: Start your reps for this exercise at the bottom position to mid point lower then curl all the way up to start position. That's one rep. Perform 12 reps total 3 sets

Resisted Pressdown (Isolation) Long head

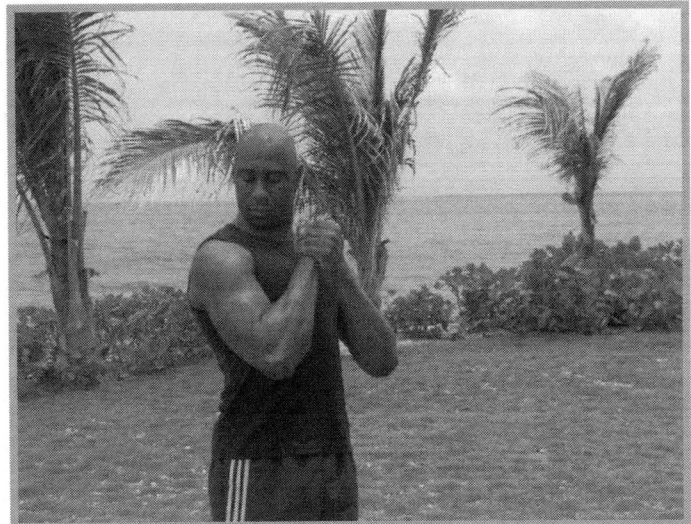

Start Position

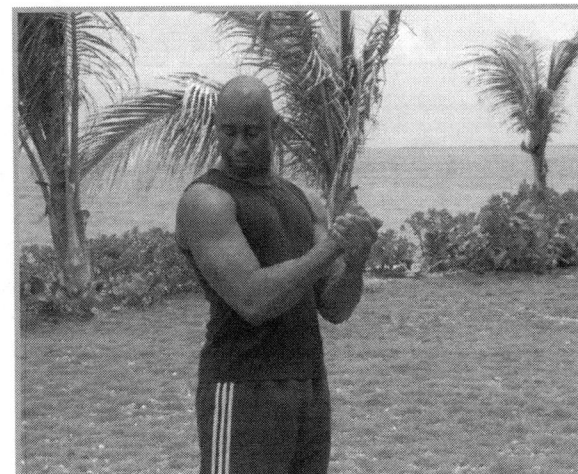

Mid-Point

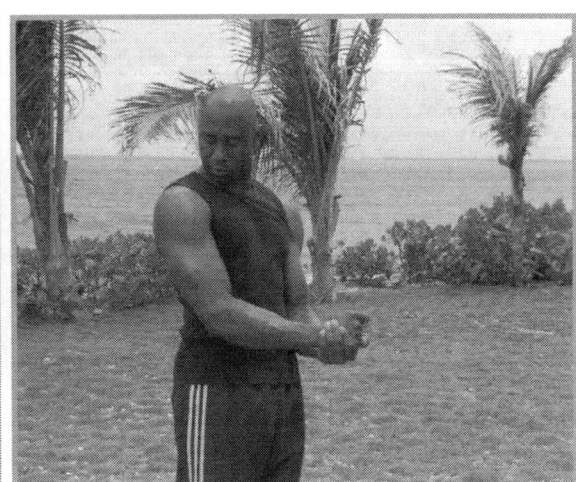

Finished Position

Double Impact Method: Start your reps for this exercise at the top position press the arm all the way down, come up half way press down. Then start all over again for 12 reps 3 sets. Then switch arms

Perform these exercises with full range no half moves 3 sets of 15 reps each. One exercise after the other until all the exercises are done.

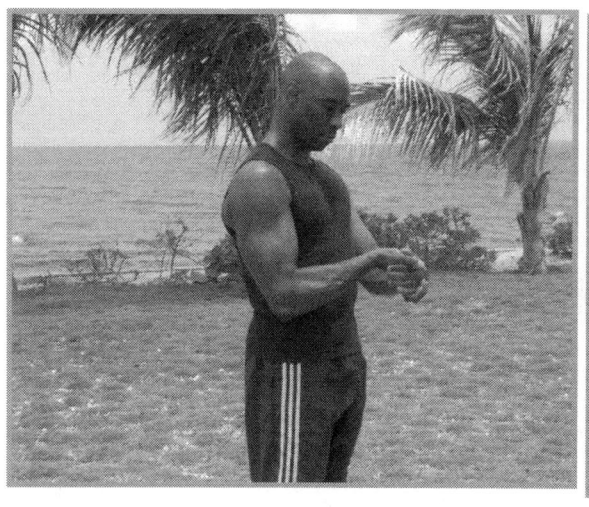
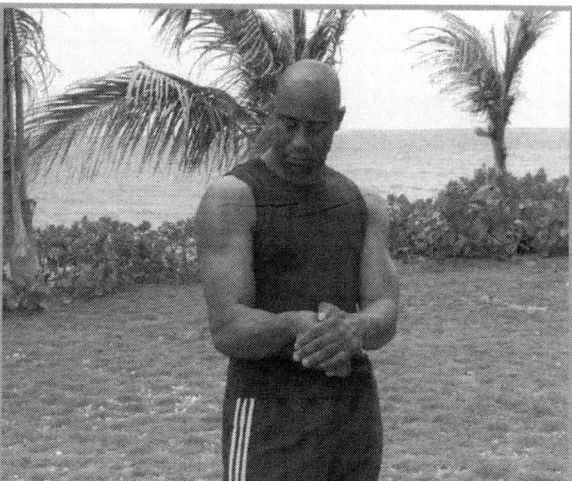
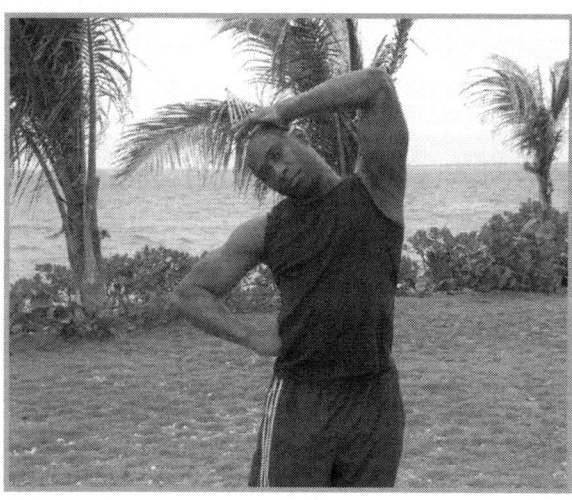
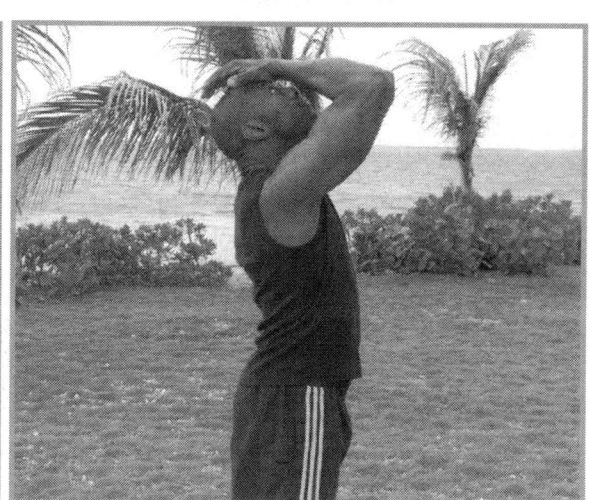
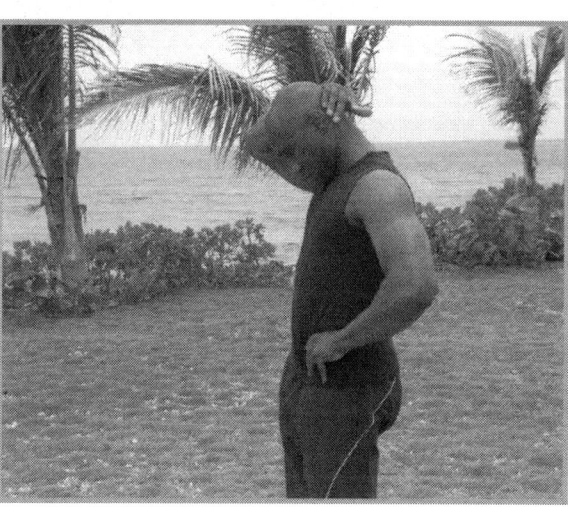
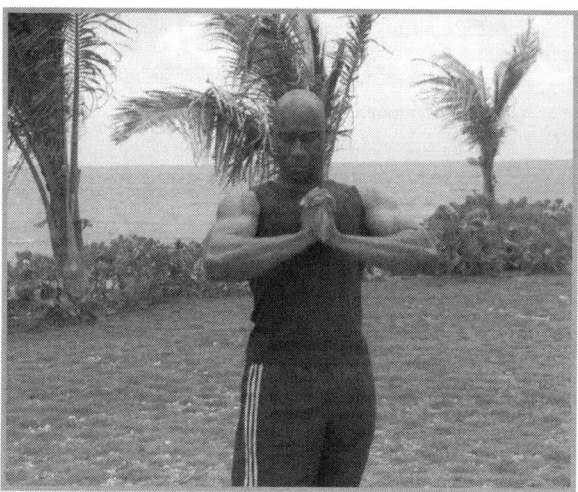

Remember Perform these exercises one after the other without rest until you've completed one full round. That's one set. 3 sets of 15 reps 3 rounds.

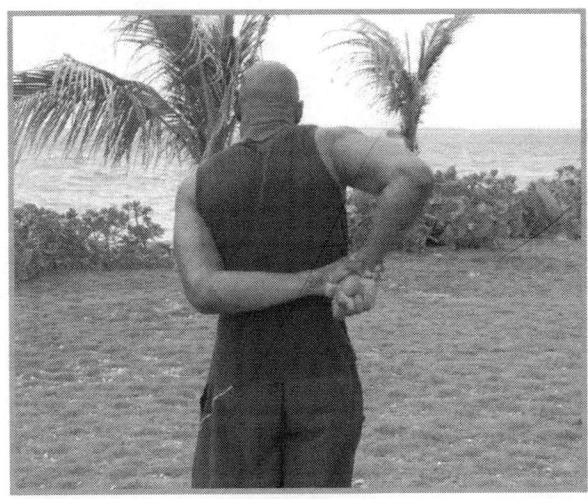
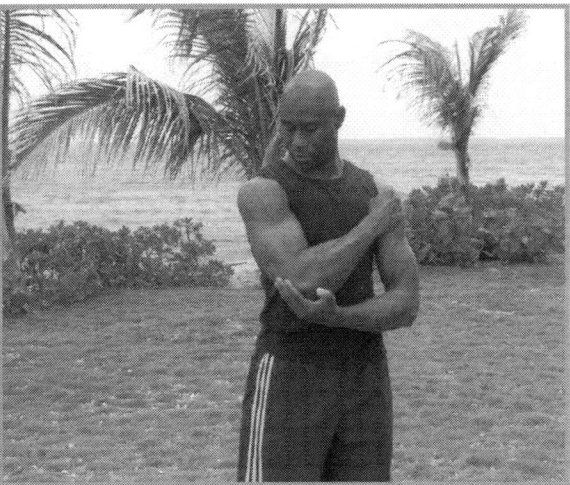
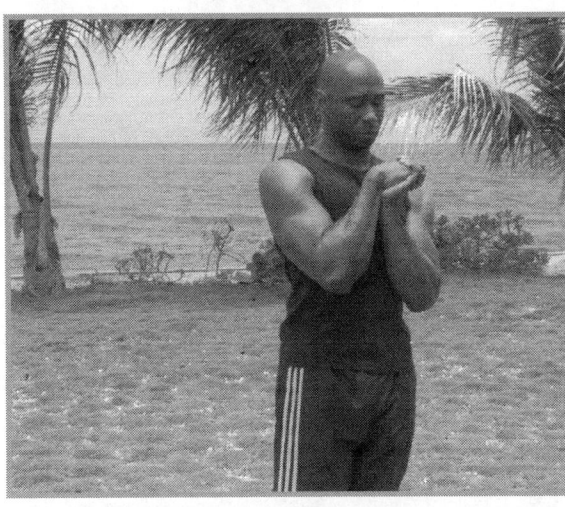
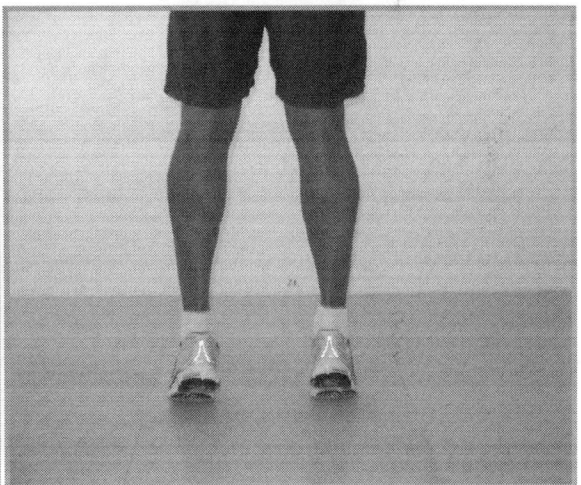
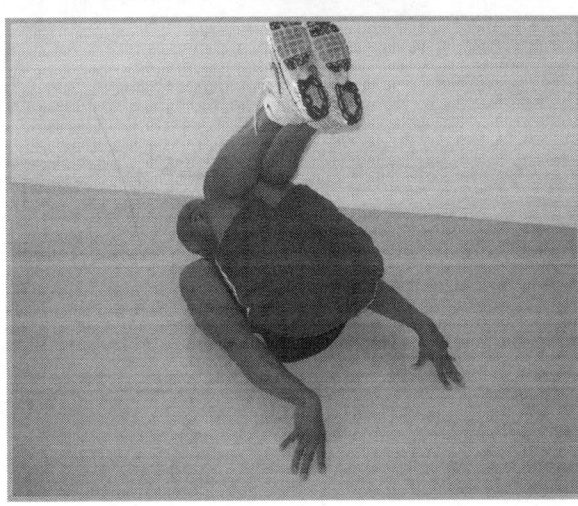

Workout Two

Double Impact Method

Workout Two

Tuesday Thursday Saturday

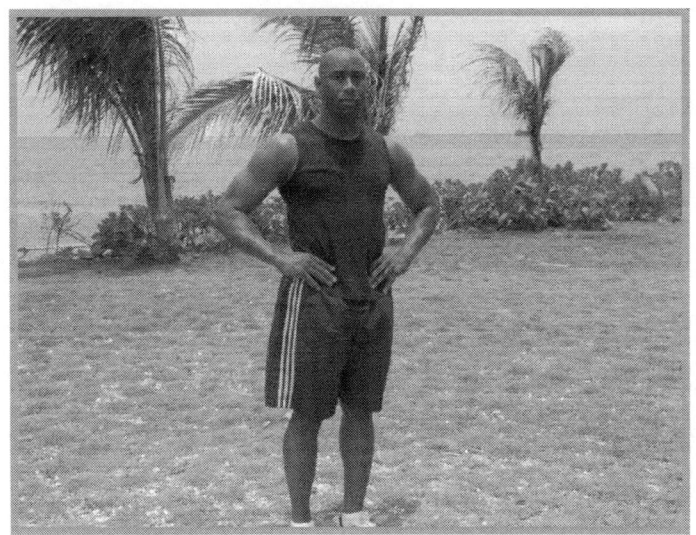

Start Position

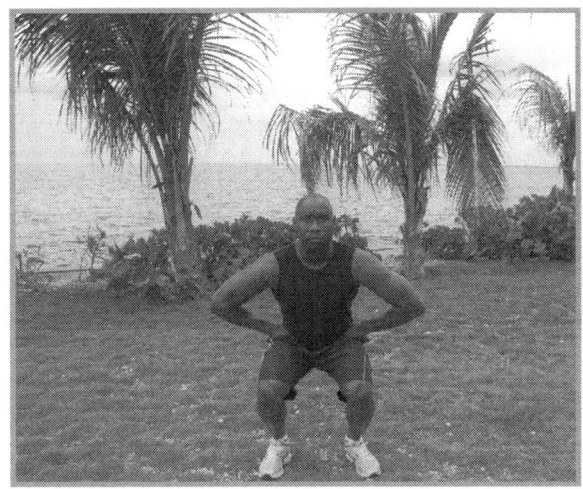

Mid-Point

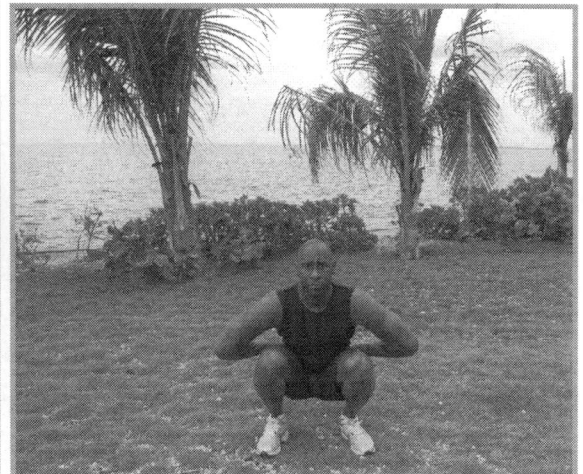

Finished Position

Double Impact Method: Start your reps for this exercise at the bottom position to mid point lower then press all the way up to start position. That's one rep. Perform 15 reps total 3 sets

Crossed Feet Squats

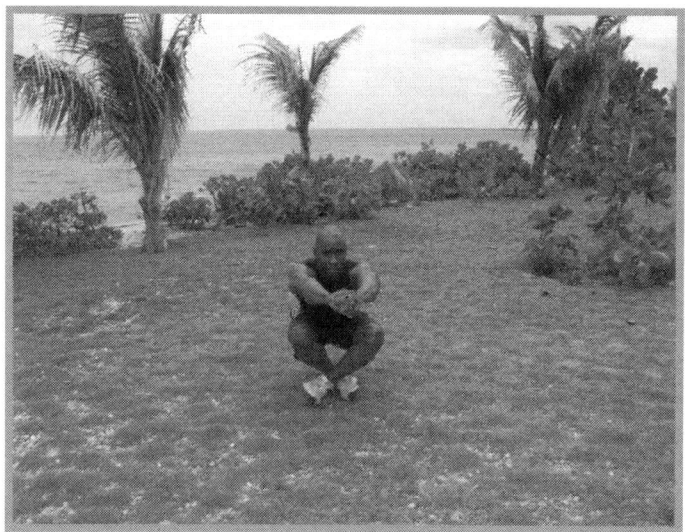

Start Position

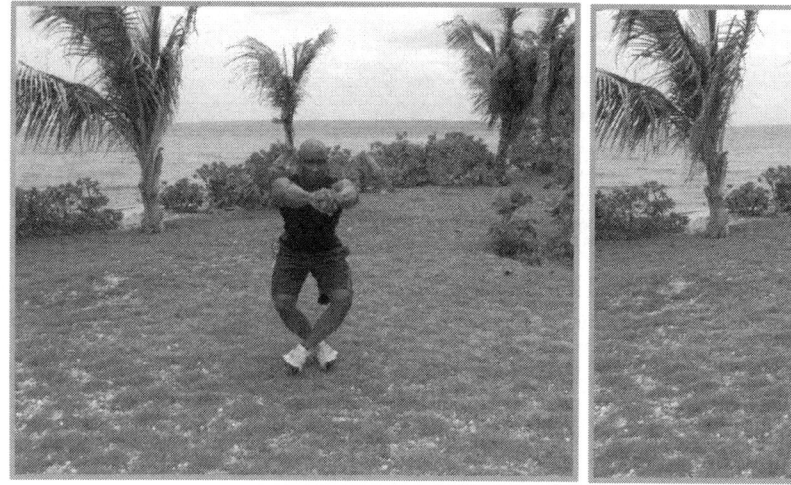

Mid-Point

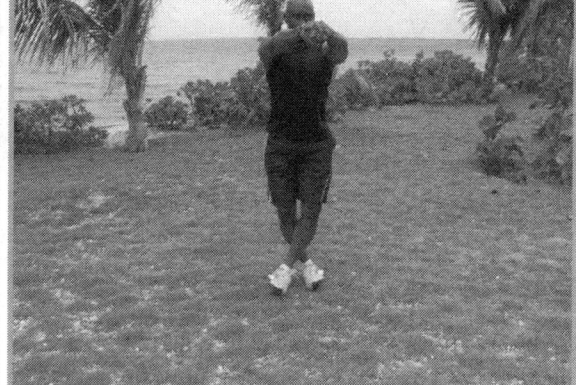

Finished Position

Double Impact Method: Start your reps for this exercise at the bottom position to mid point lower then press all the way up to start position. That's one rep. Perform 12 reps total 3 sets

Seated Resisted Leg Curls

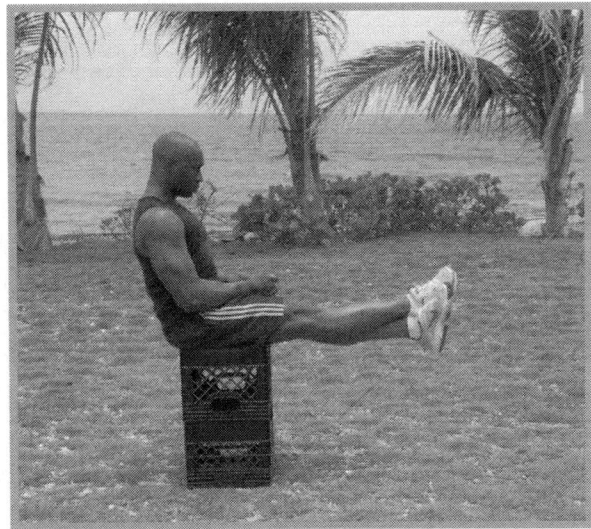

Start Position

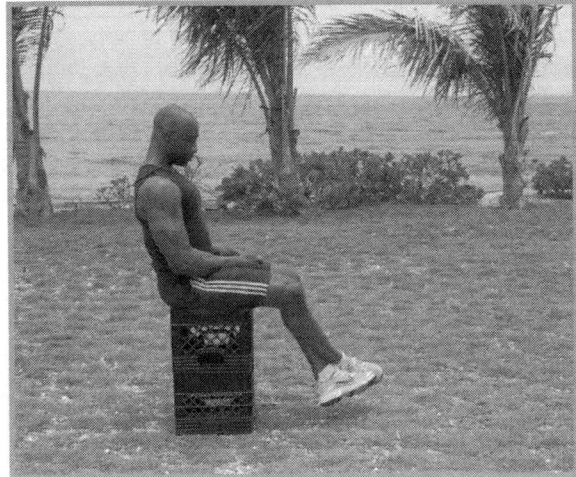

Mid-Point

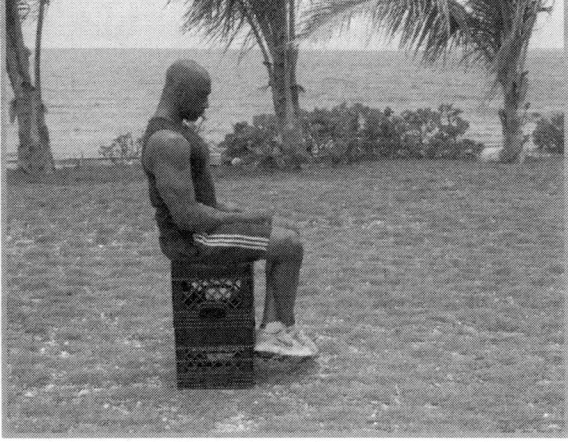

Finished Position

Double Impact Method: Start the exercise at the start position shown, perform a full rep followed by a half rep at the mid point. Then start at the top position again. 12 reps total 3 sets each leg.

Perform these exercises one after the other until all the exercises are completed in one set (round) Perform 3 sets of 15-20 reps each exercise full reps.

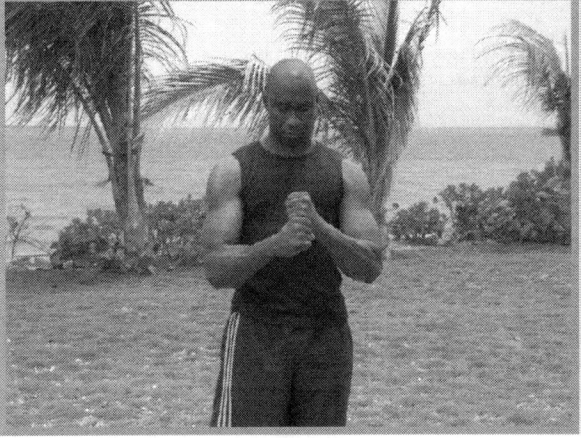
Neutral Hammer Curls

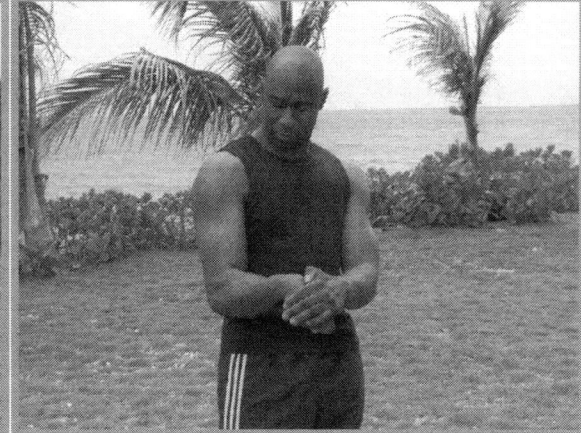
Reverse Wrist Curls

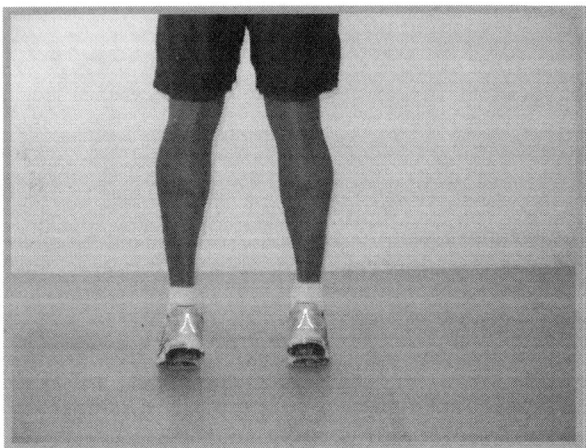
Standing Calve Raises

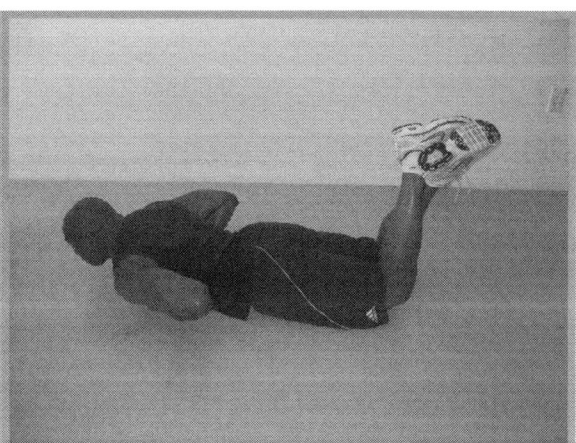
Lying Leg Curls

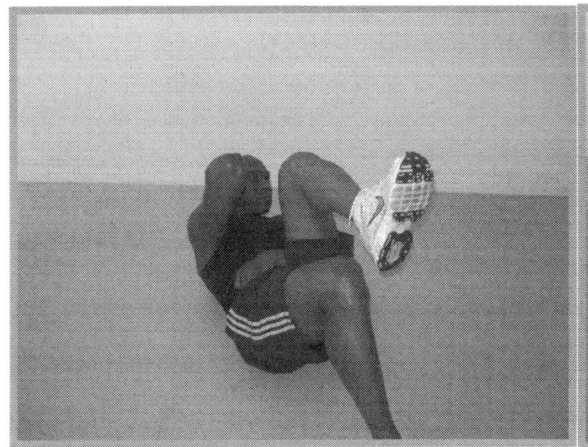
Side Crunches

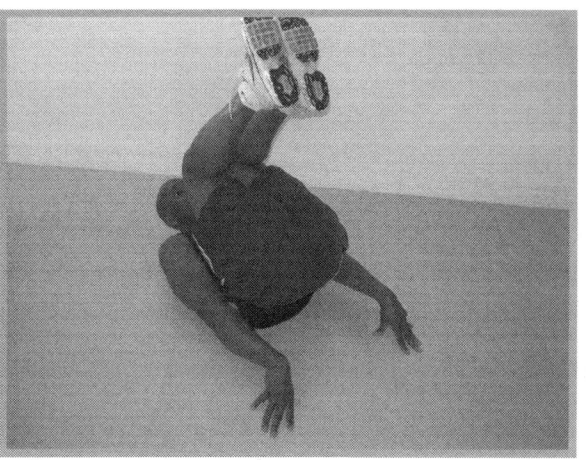
Reverse Crunches

Perform these exercises one after the other until all the exercises are completed in one set (round) Perform 3 sets of 15-20 reps each exercise full reps

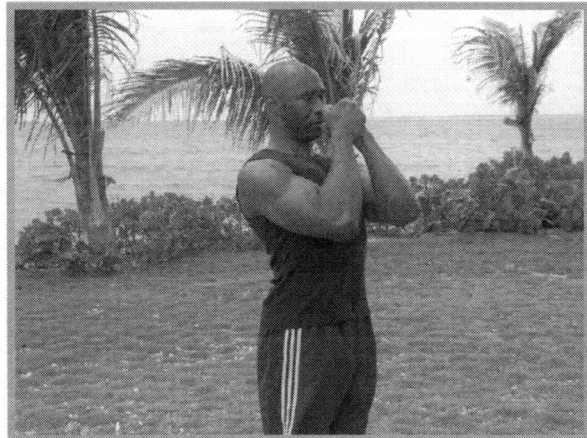
Forward Extensions

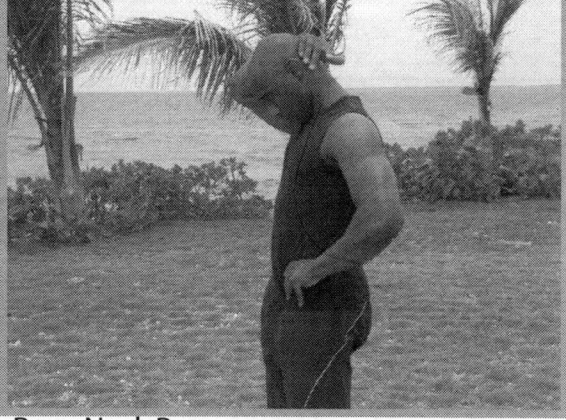
Rear Neck Press

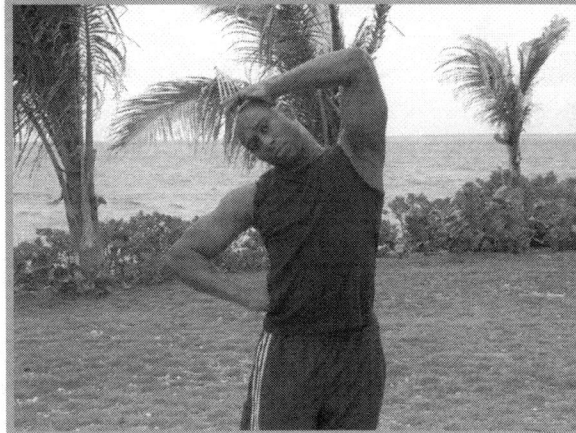
Side Neck Press

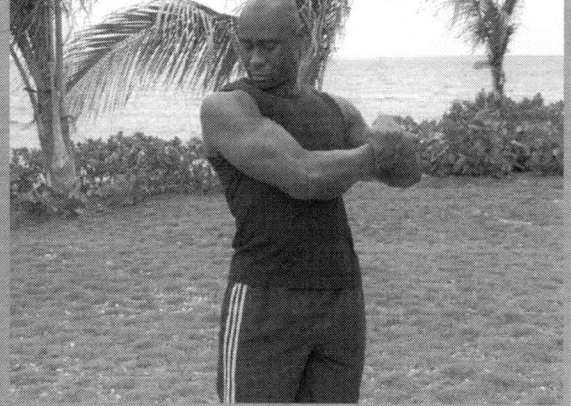
Across-The-Body-Pulls

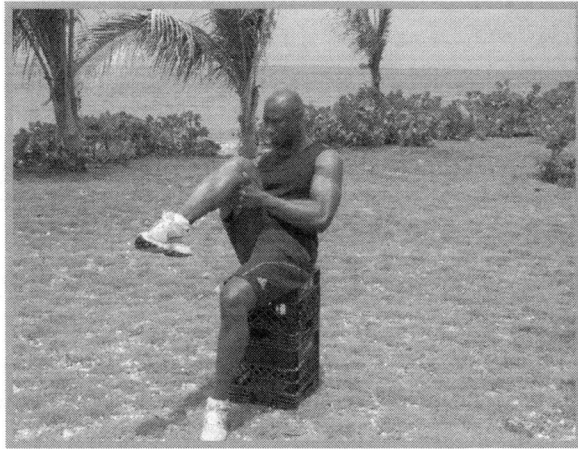
Seated Thigh Rows

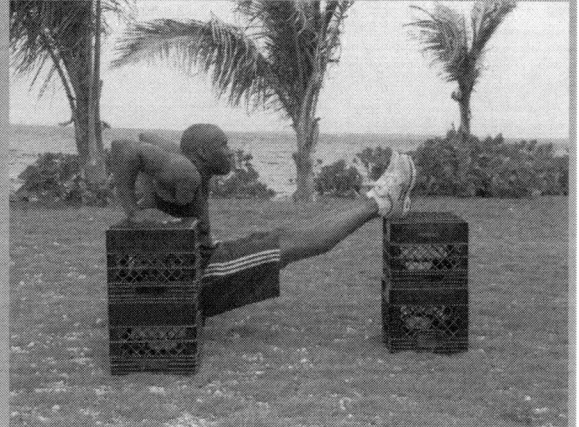
Three-Chair-Dips

Chapter 6

*Compound Isolation Training Routine
One Phase Three Perform for 3 weeks*

CHAPTER 6

Routine One Compound Isolation Training   Chest

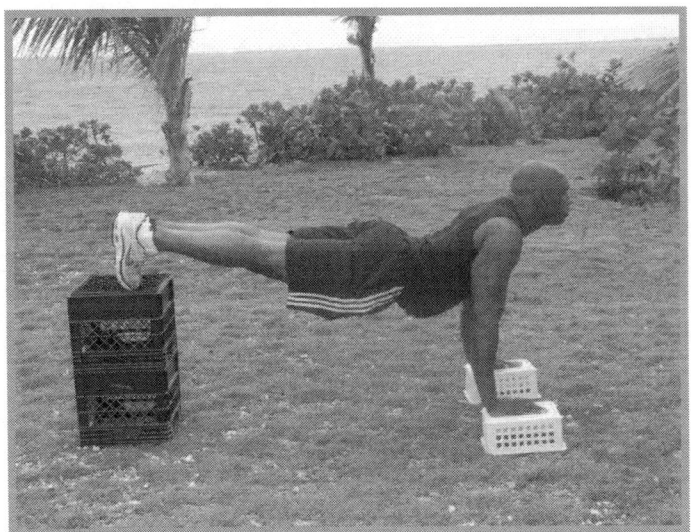

Decline Pushups

Perform 2-3 sets full reps pausing at the bottom to pre-stretch the chest before pressing upwards again.

SUPERSET THESE TWO EXERCISES

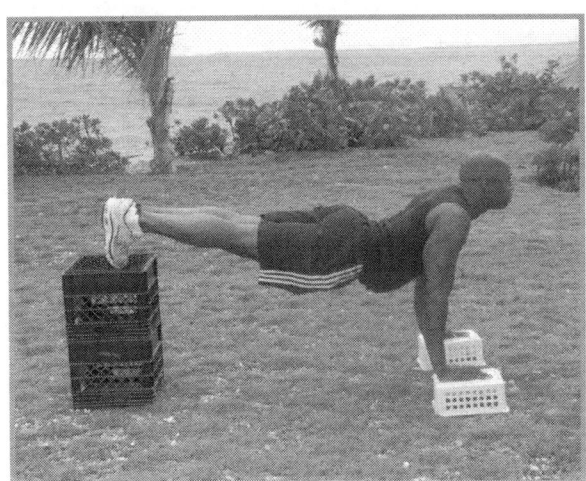 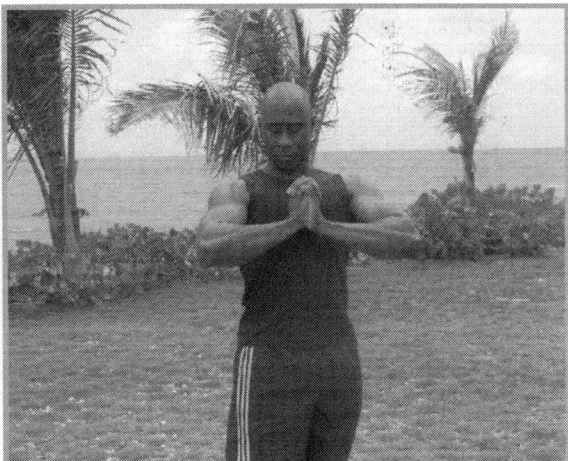

Decline Pushups   Liederman Presses

Remember to pause at the bottom of the pushups to pre-stretch the chest for added growth. Also pause on the liedermans at the shoulder before reversing the exercise. Perform 12-15 reps each exercise at 2-3 sets each

Back

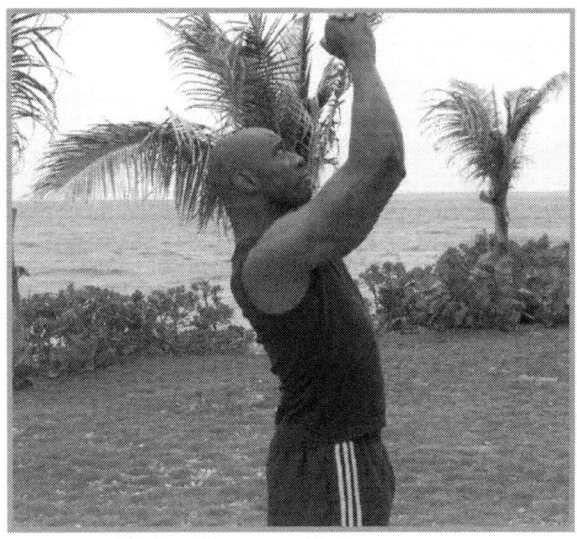 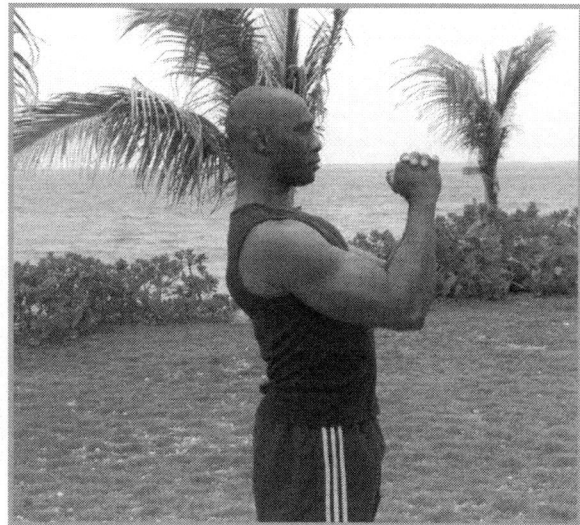

Start Position   Finished Position

Perform 12 reps each arm (resisting both ways) 3 sets each side.

SUPERSET THESE TWO EXERCISES

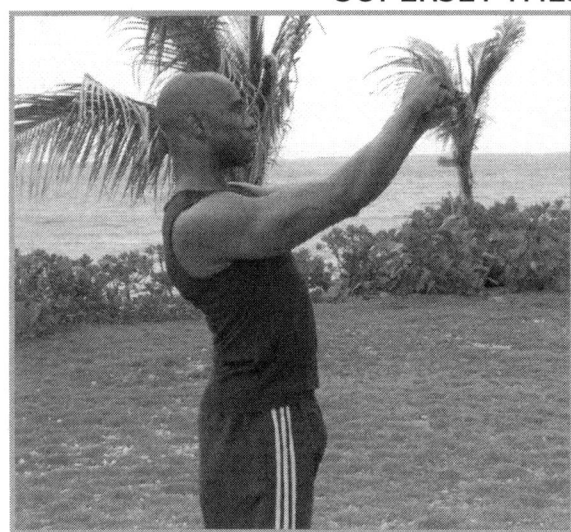 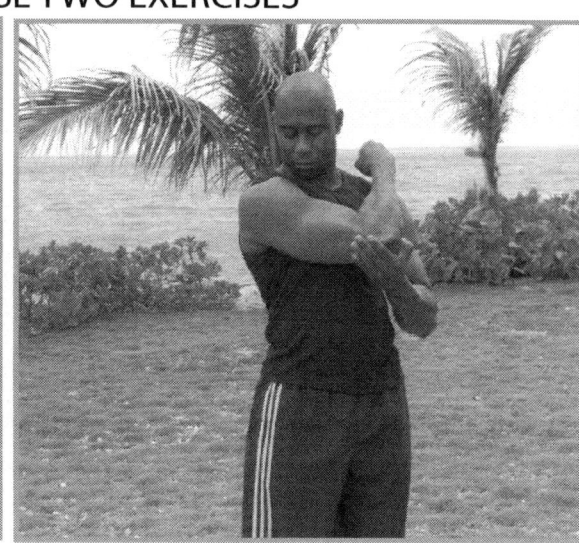

Stiff Arm Pulldowns   Across-The-Body Pulls

Work the right side of both exercises first before moving to the left side. Perform 3 sets 12 reps each side.

Biceps/Forearms

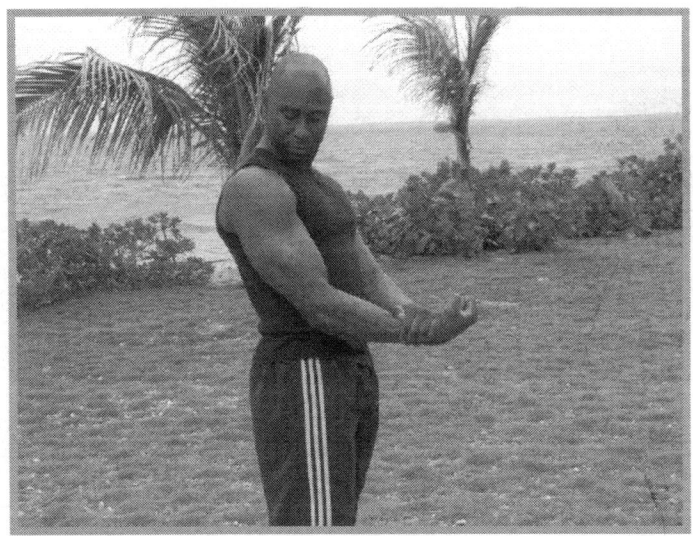

Perform 12-15 reps at 3 sets per arm.

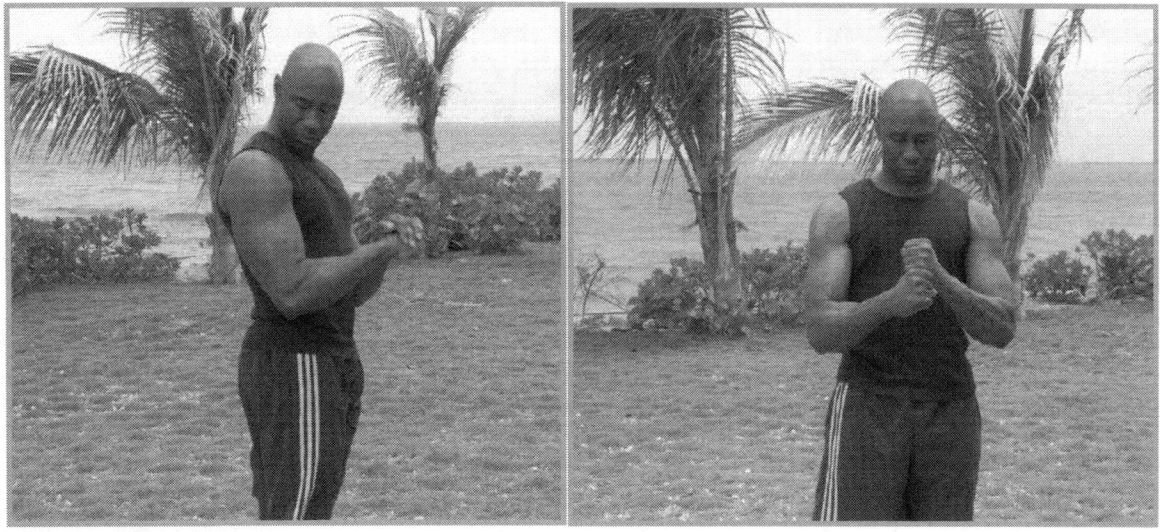

Reverse Curls   Hammer Curls

Perform 12 reps of the two exercises without rest, then switch arms and repeat. 3 sets each.

Forearms   Palm Up and Palm Down Wrist Curls

SUPERSET THESE TWO EXERCISES

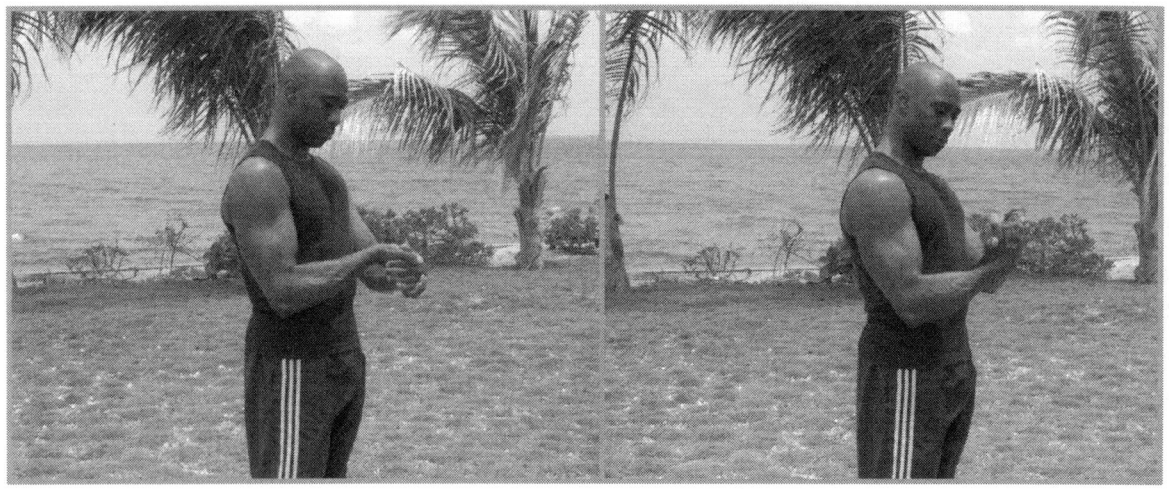

Start Position   Finished Position

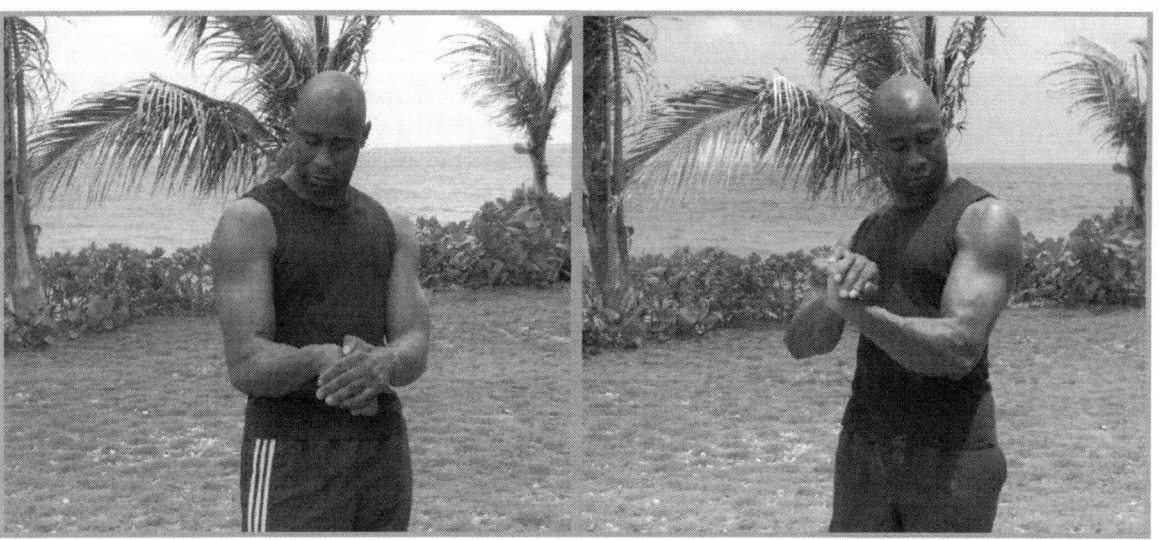

Start Position   Finished Position

Perform the superset on right forearm first before switching to the left forearm for another superset. 15-20 reps at 3-4 sets

ABS

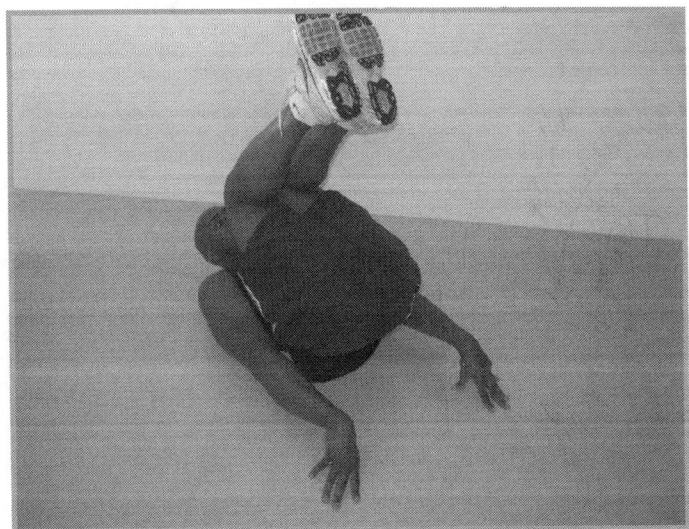

Reverse Crunches (Basic)

15-20 reps at 3-4 sets is where it's at with this exercise.

Side Crunches

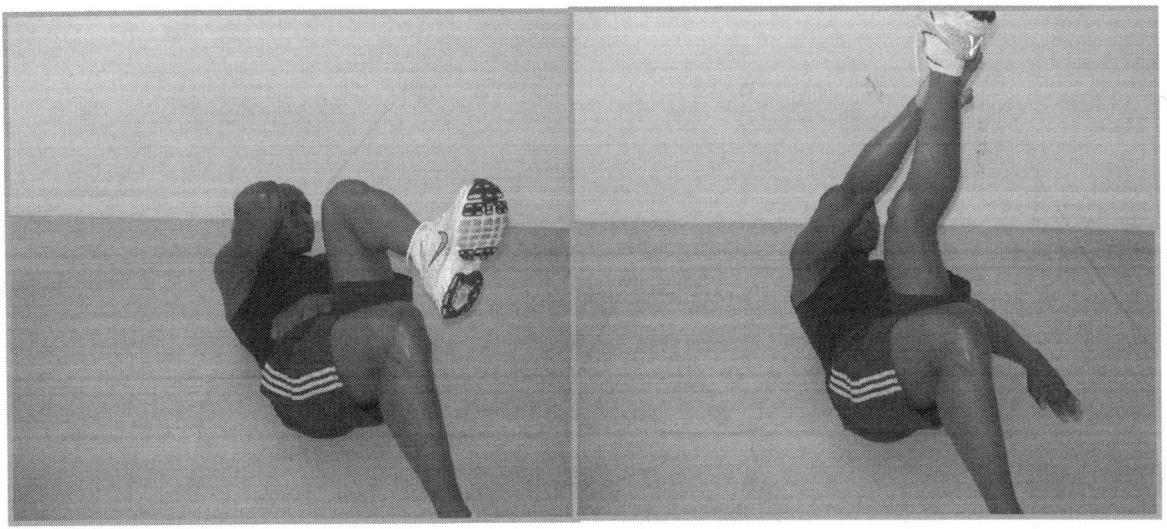

Bent Knee   Extended Version

Again 15-20 reps are perfect at 4 sets. This is another variation worth a try when variety is needed. Awesome for obliques.

Calve Superset

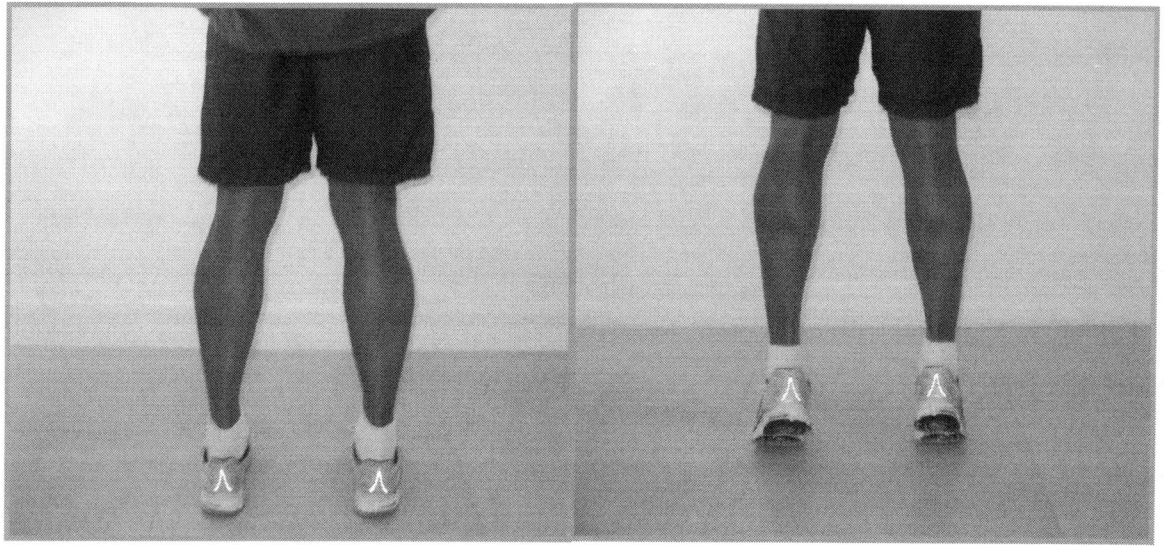

Start Position   Finished Position

Standing and Slanted Calve Raises

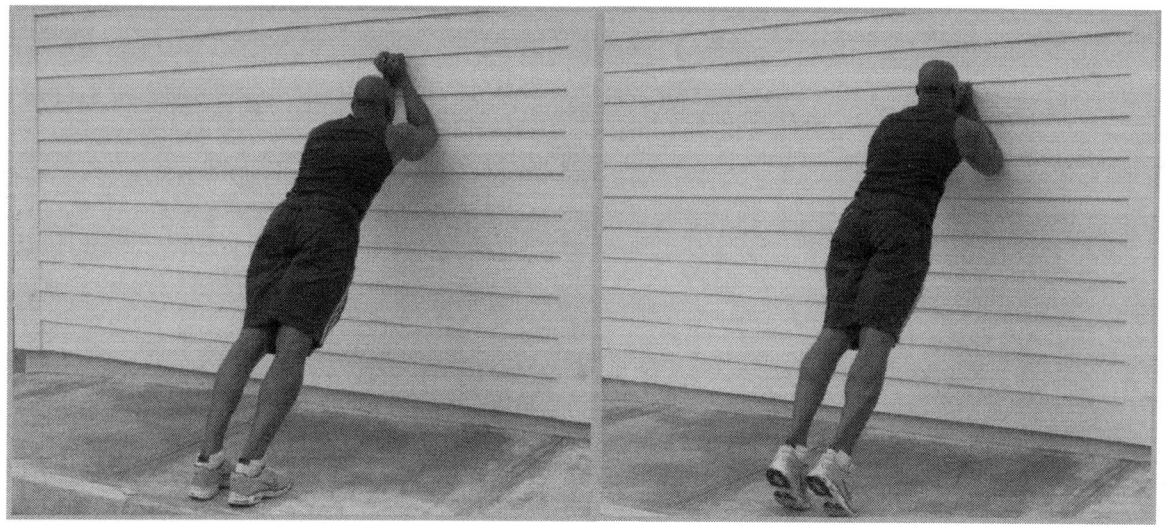

Start Position   Finished Position

Standing Calve raises can be performed at the edge of a staircase to pre-stretch the calves further. 20-25 reps each exercise is enough stimulation for this superset.

WorkOut Two   Tuesday, Thursday and Saturdays

Shoulders
Decline Pushups

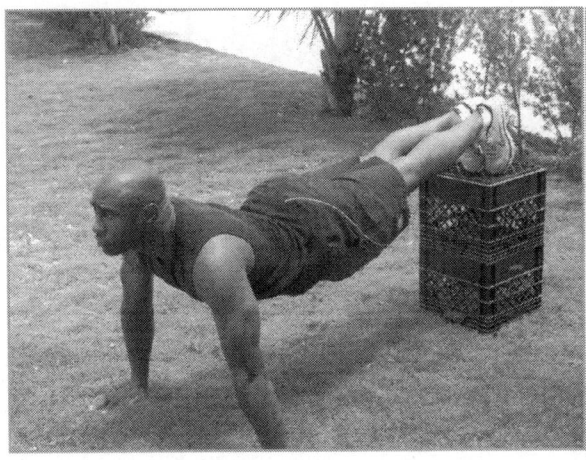
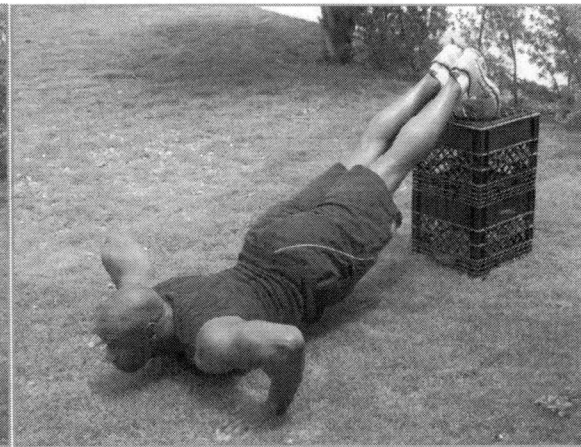

Start Position   Finished Position

12-15 reps at 3-4 sets Max!

SUPERSET THESE TWO EXERCISES

Resisted Upright Pulls

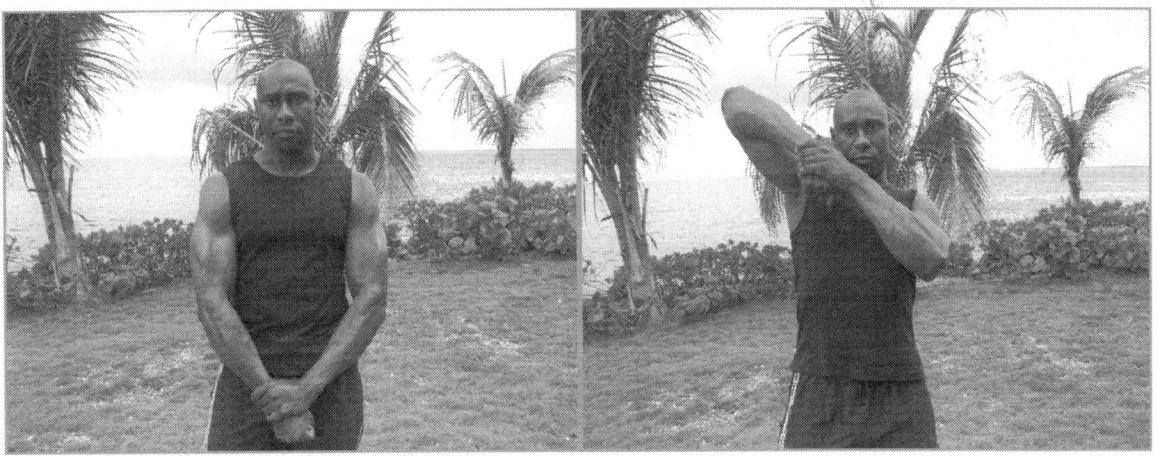

Start Position   Finished Position

Superset Workout Continued...

Across the body Lateral Raises

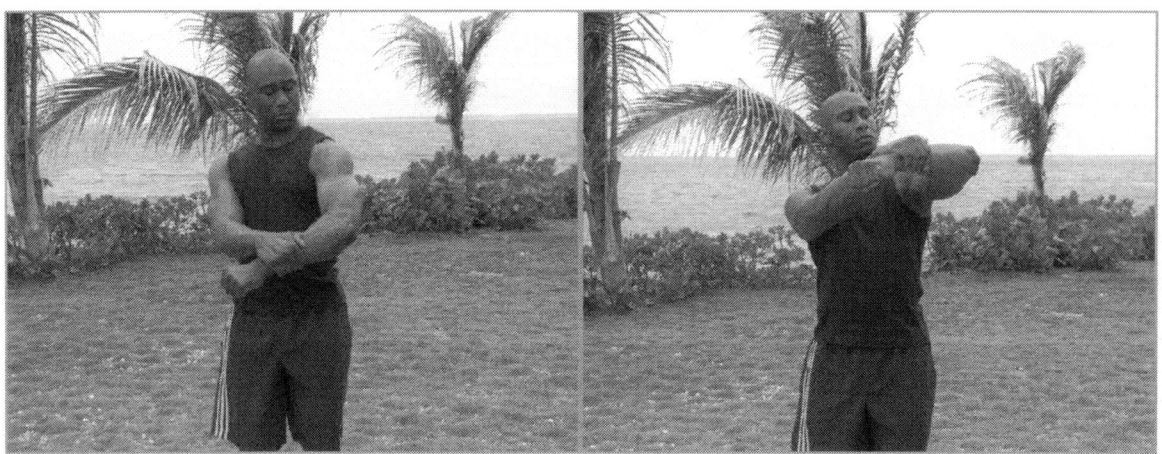

Start Position   Finished Position

Perform the superset on one side first before switching to the other arm. 12-15 reps each arm at 3-4 sets is enough.

SUPERSET THESE TWO EXERCISES

Resisted Forward Raises

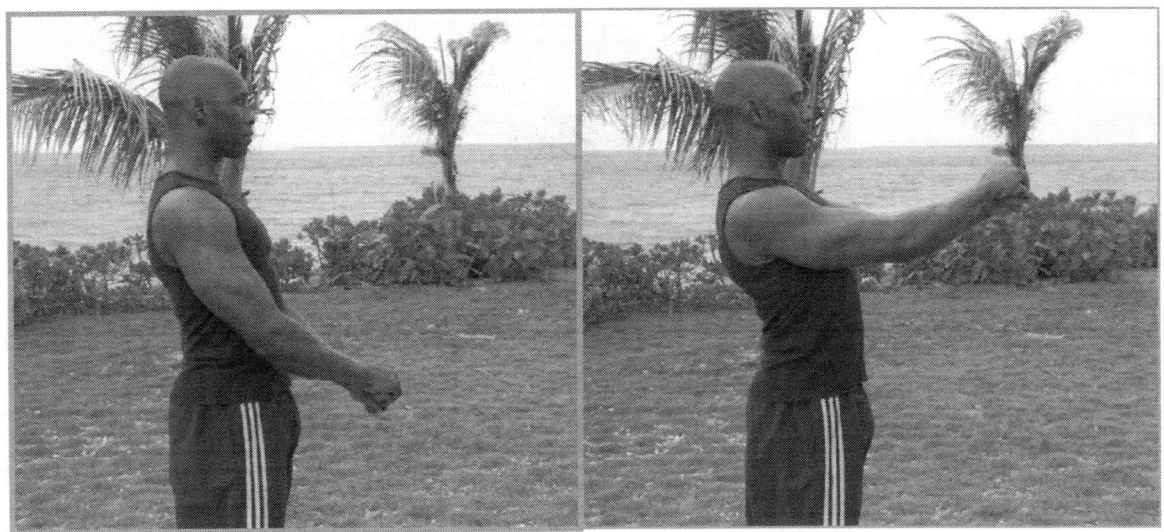

Start Position   Finished Position

Resisted Shoulder Press

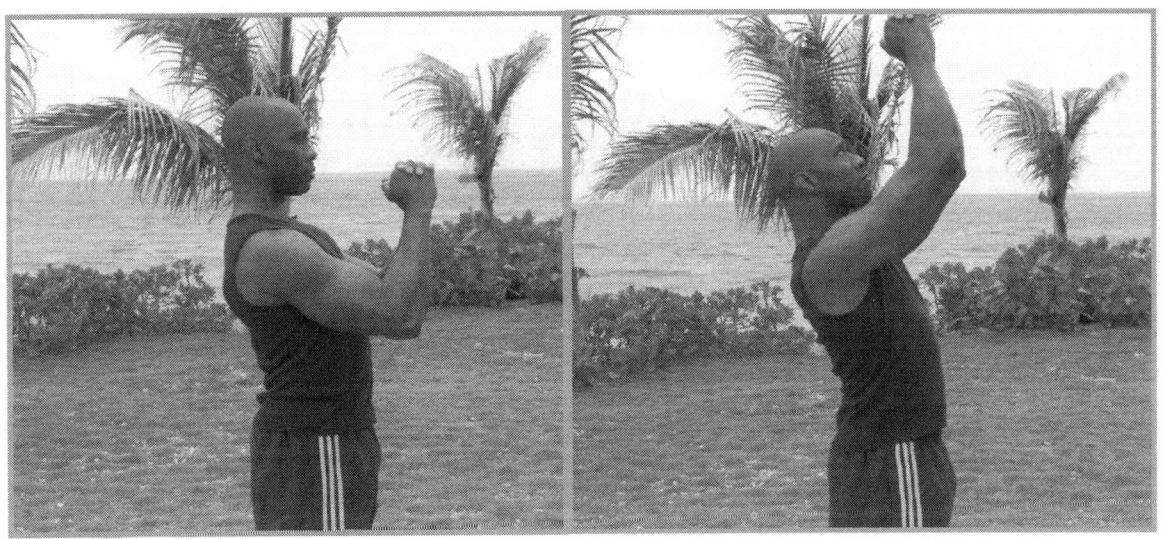

Start Position   Finished Position

Perform the right arm superset first before proceeding to the left. 15 reps at 3 sets is perfect!

Triceps

Decline Tricep Extensions (Basic)

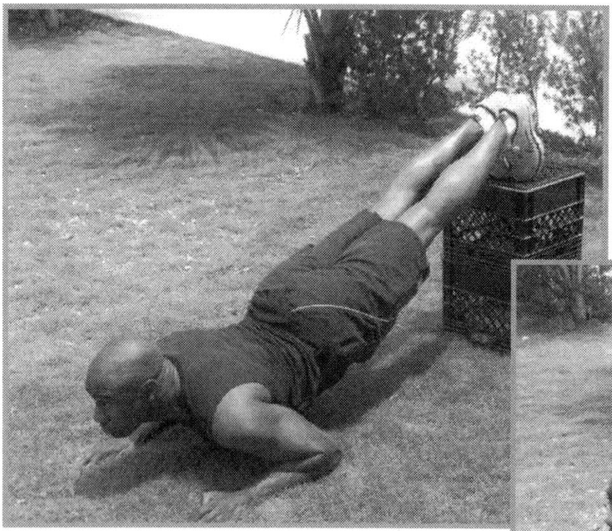

Start Position
Perform 7-9 reps at 3 sets.
Keep the elbows bent on the way up.

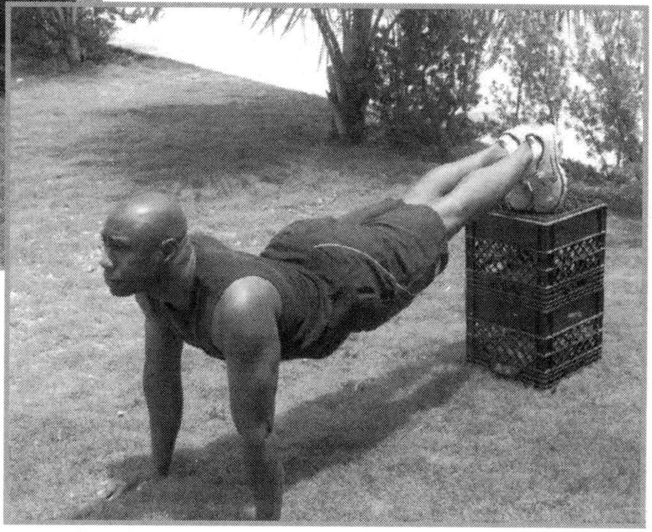

Finished Position

SUPERSET THESE TWO EXERCISES

Tricep Pressdowns

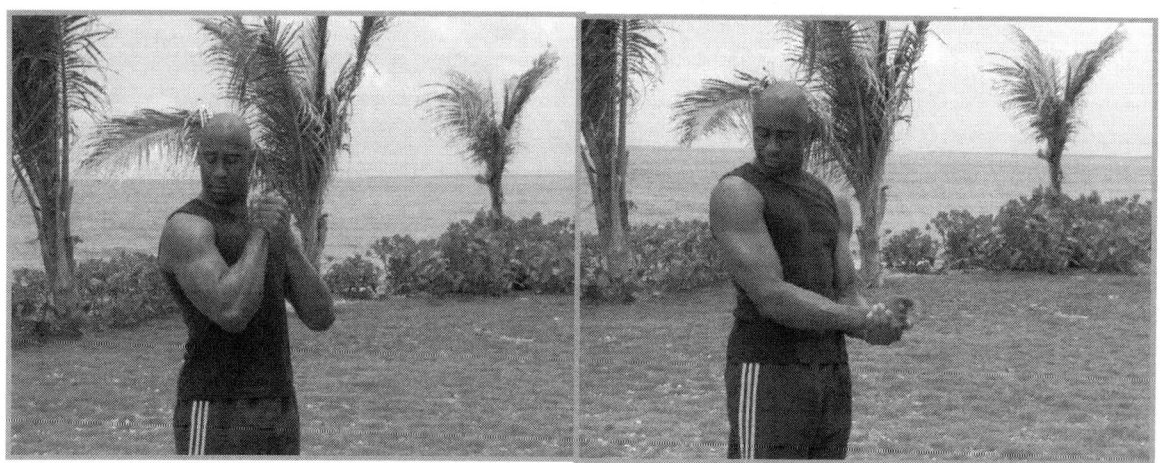

Superset Workout Continued...

Tricep Forward Extension

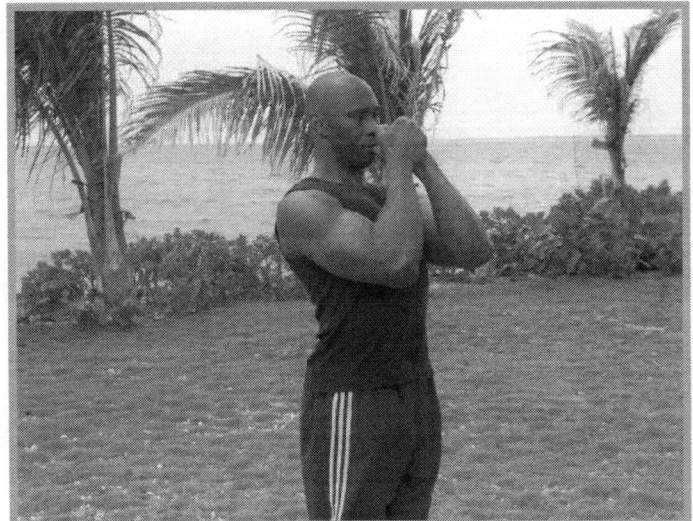

Start Position

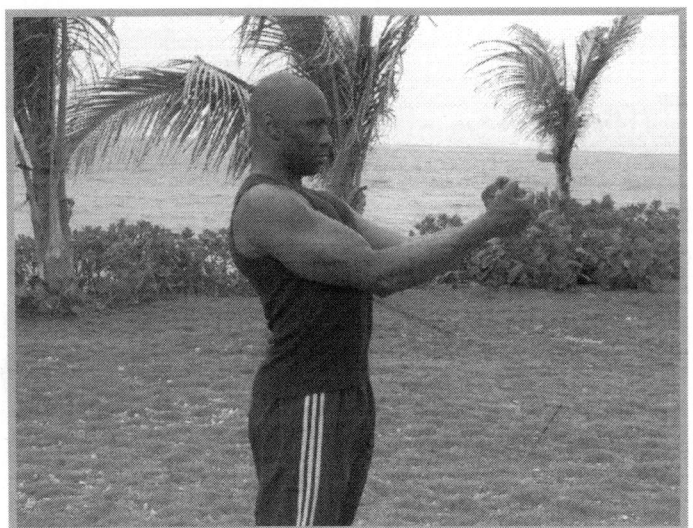

Finished Position

12-15 reps per side at 3 sets are Best!

Squats (Basic)

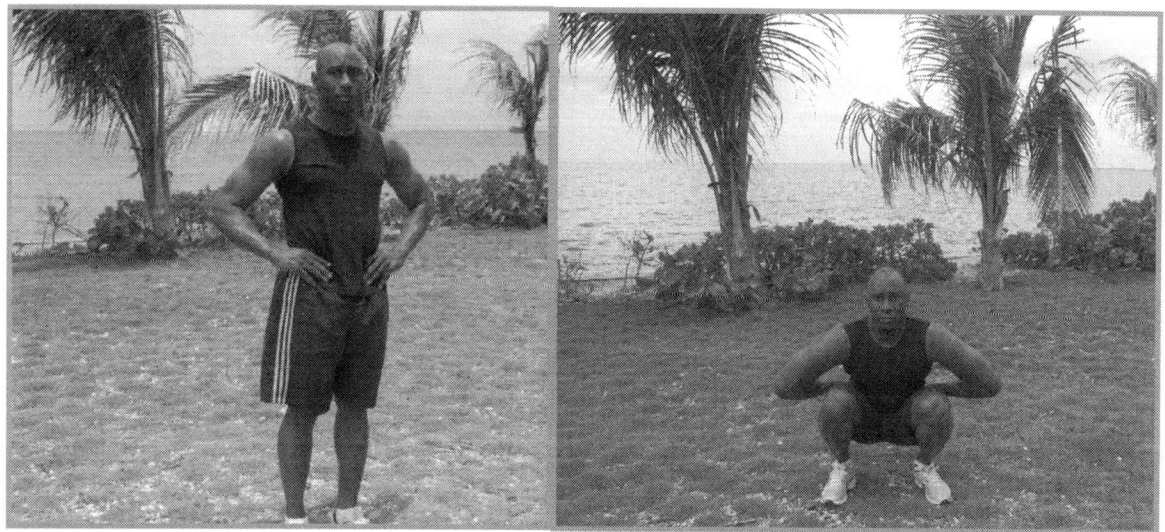

Start Position   Finished Position

The Squat the King of all lower body exercises. 20 reps of 3 sets are enough.

SUPERSET THESE TWO EXERCISES

Crossed Feet Squats

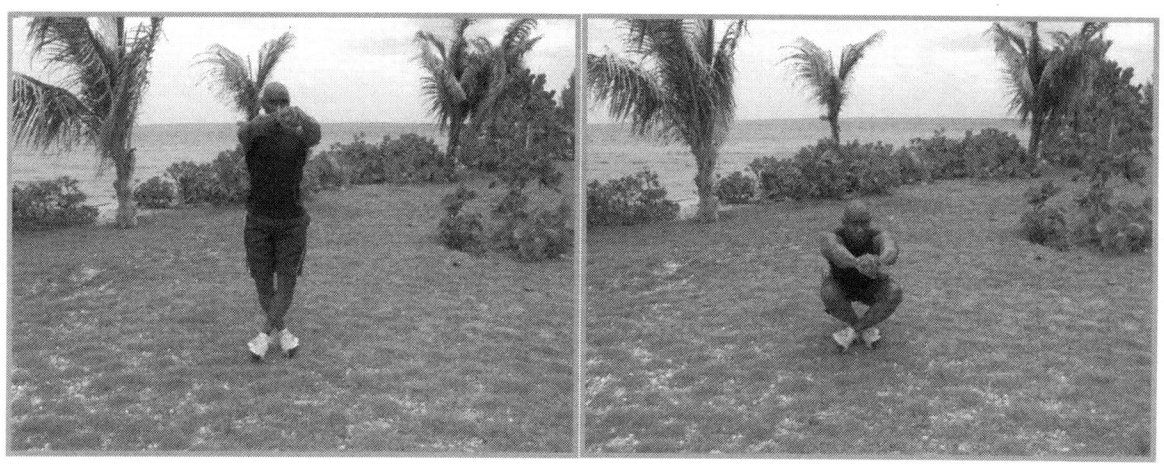

Start Position   Finished Position

Superset Workout Continued....

Regular Squats

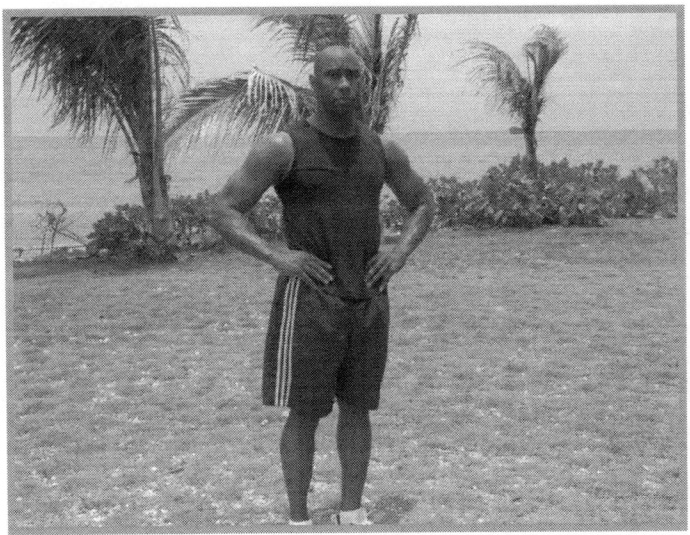

Start Position

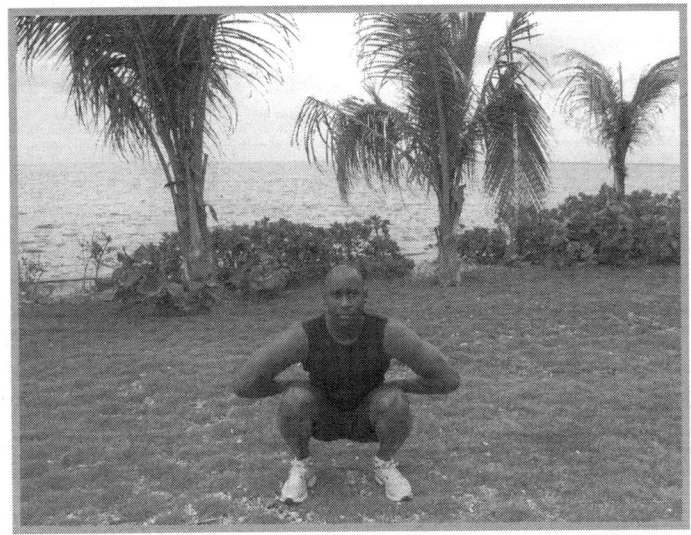

Finished Position

20-25 reps each superset at 3-4 sets are enough to stimulate all the muscle fibers and add strength to the hips.

Hamstrings

SUPERSET THESE TWO EXERCISES

Leg Curls

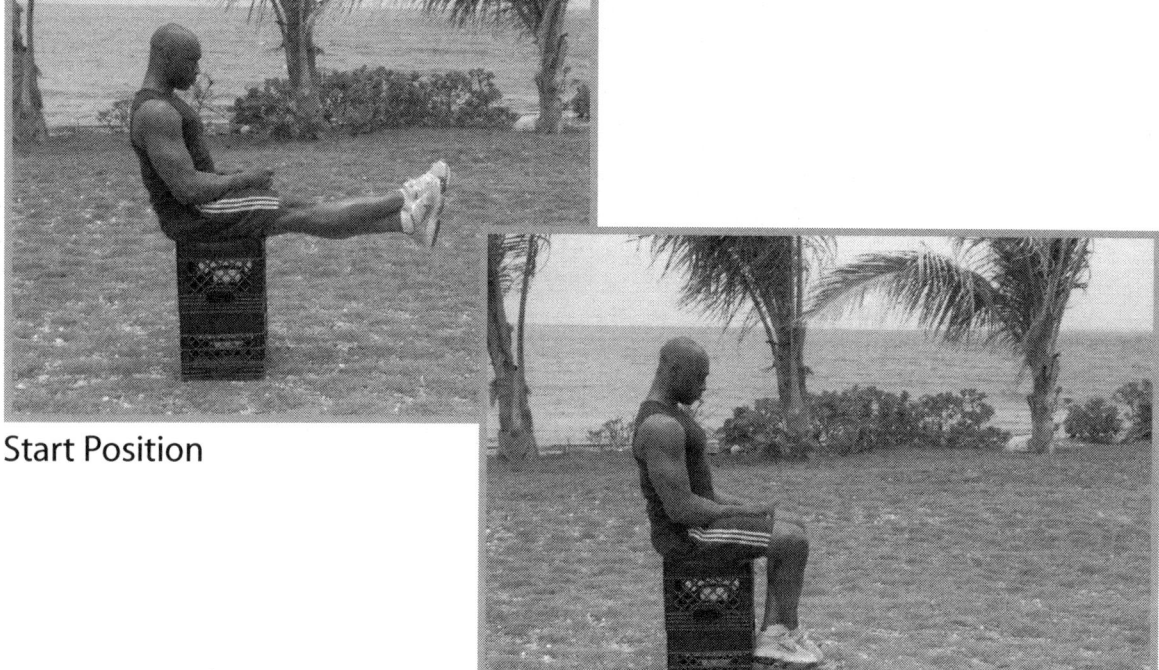

Start Position

Finished Position

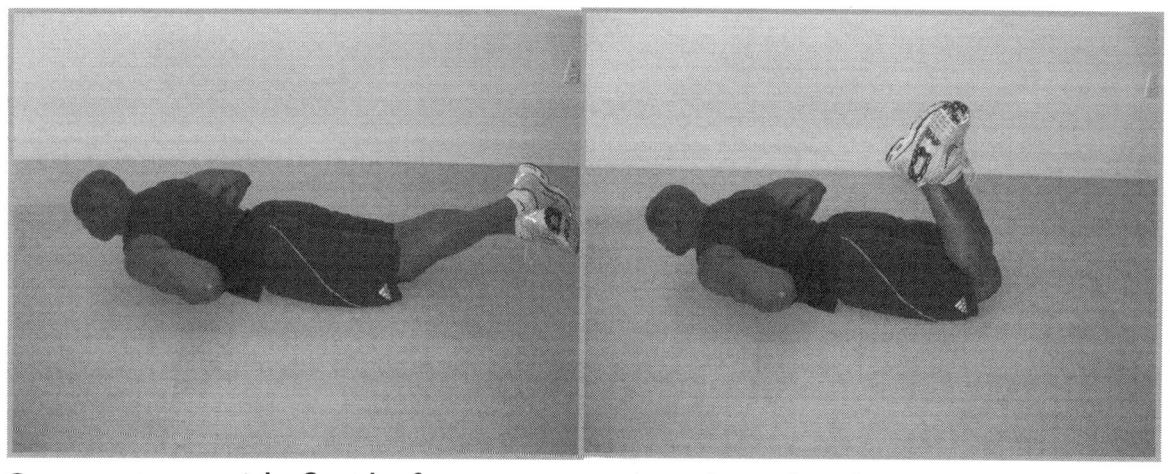

Superset one side first before supersetting the other leg. 15-20 reps at 3-4 sets are enough with these supersets.

Neck (Upper Traps) Rear Delts (Basic)

Resisted Rear Upright Pulls

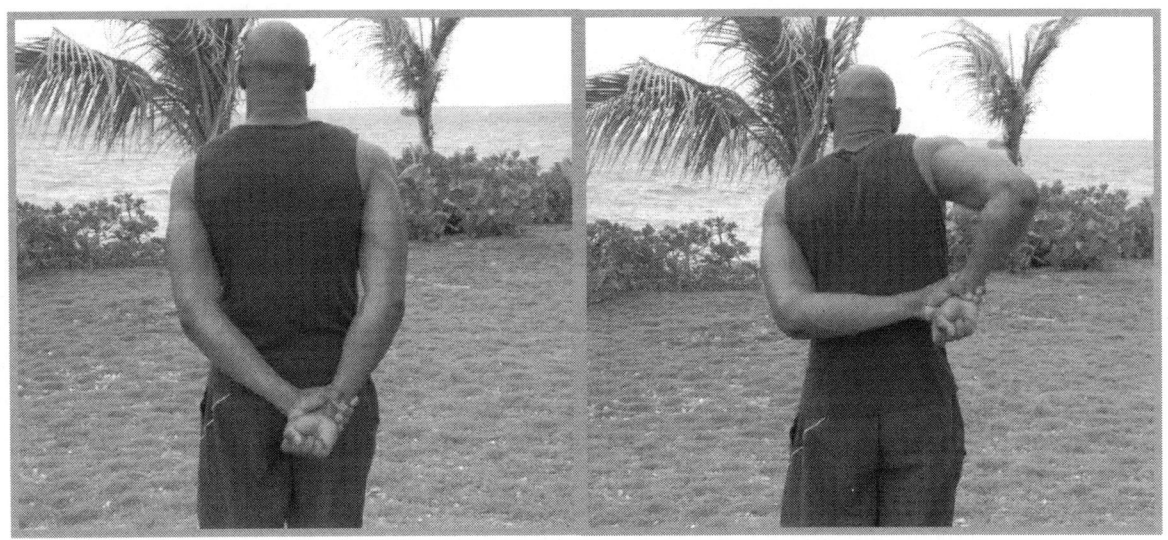

Start Position   Finished Position

Perform 15-20 reps at 3 sets each arm.

SUPERSET THESE TWO EXERCISES

Side to side Neck Press

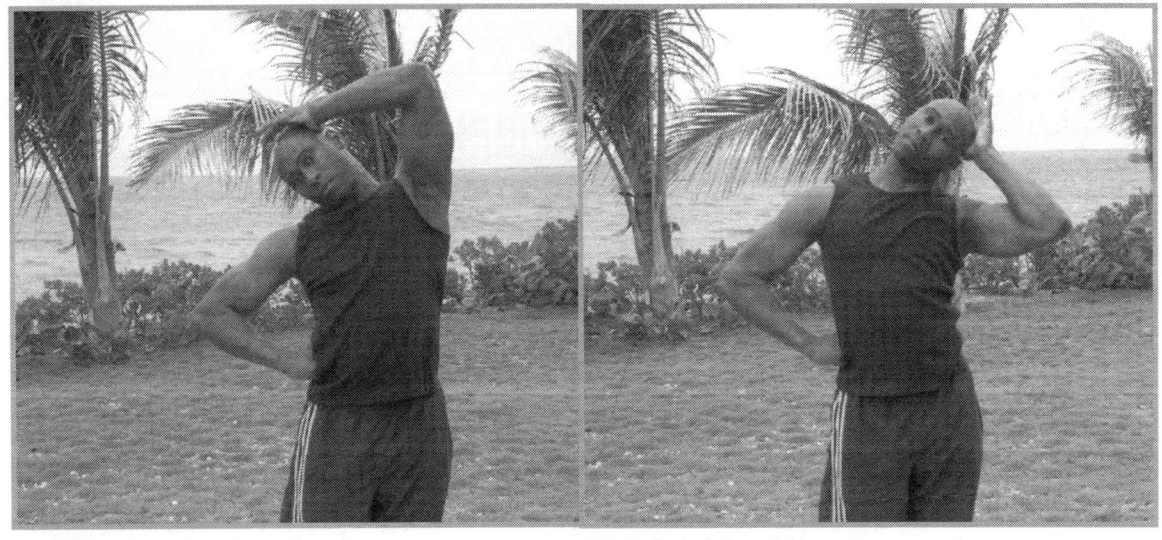

Start Position   Finished Position

Superset Workout Continued.....

Rear Neck Press

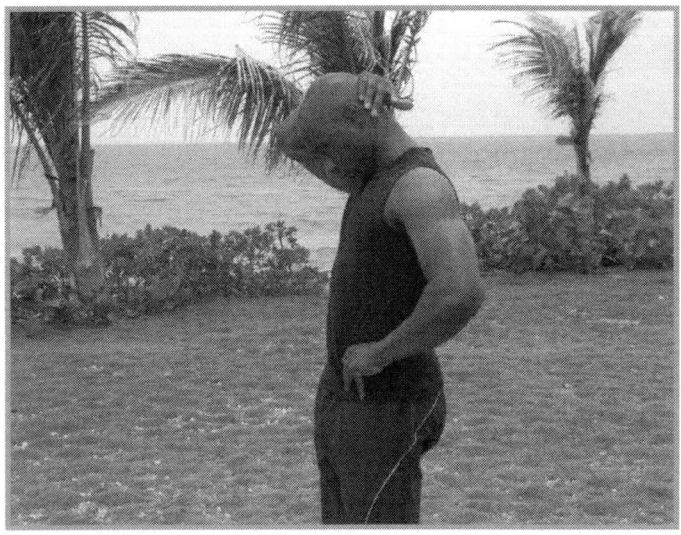

Start Position

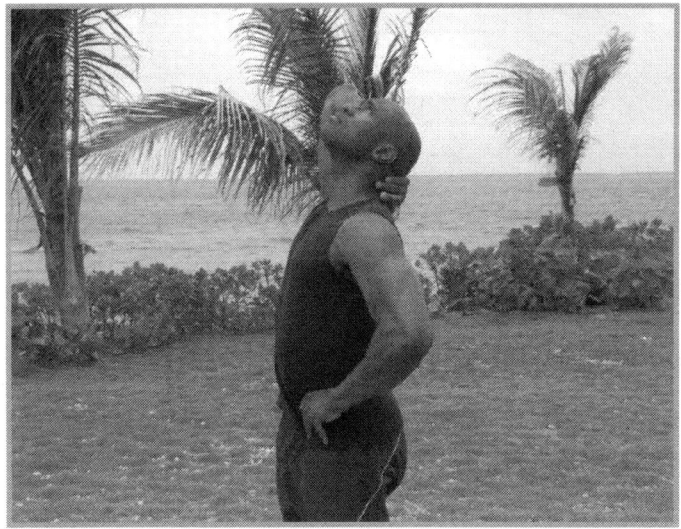

Finished Position

This superset requires 15-20 reps at 3 sets each.

Lower and Upper Back (Basic)

Thigh Rows

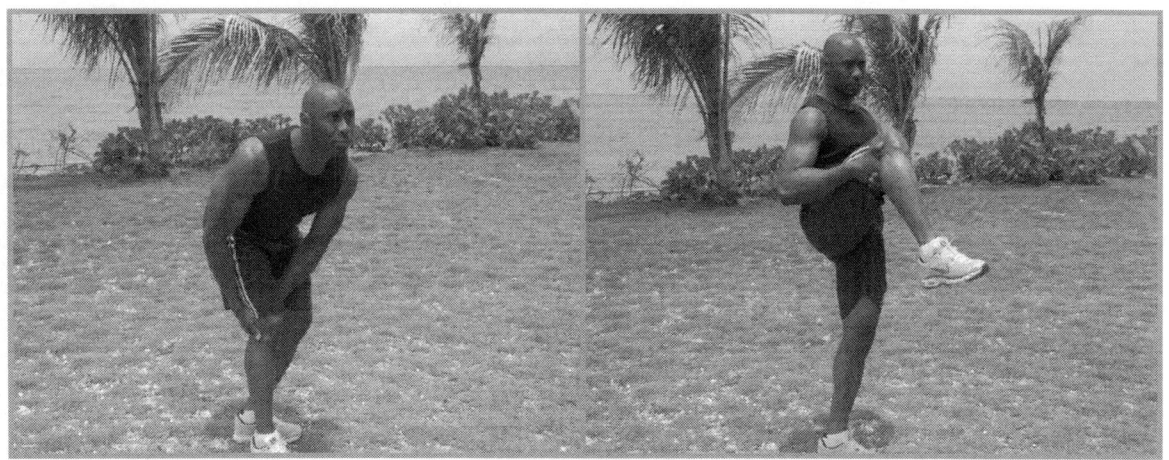

Start Position   Finished Position

If your balance isn't ideal lean against a wall. Perform 15 reps each side 3 sets each.

Forearms, Connective Tissues and Wrists

Forearm Presses

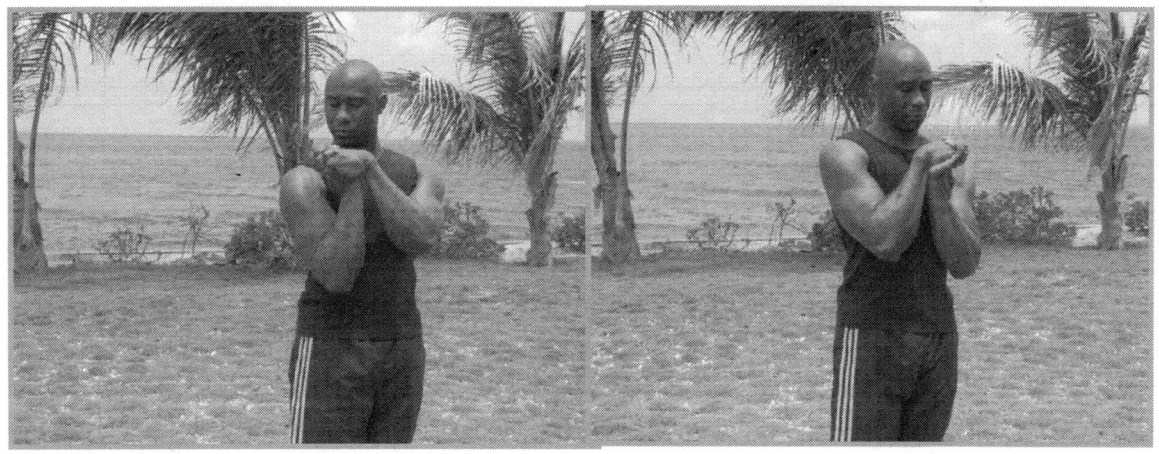

Start Position   Finished Position

20 reps of 3 sets is all that's needed for this movement for powerful forearms.

SUPERSET THESE TWO EXERCISES

Palm Up Wrist Curls

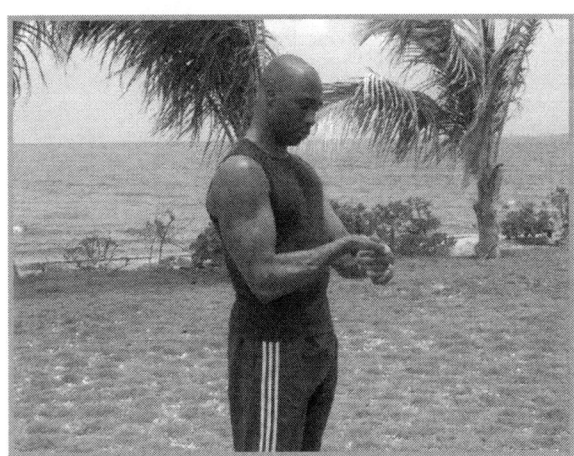

Start Position

Palm Down Wrist Curls

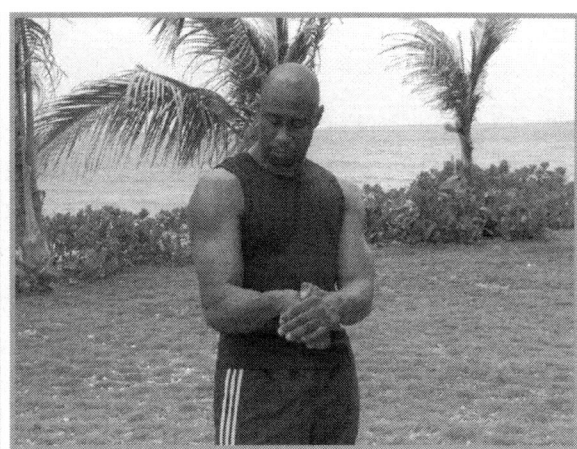

Finished Position

12-15 reps at 4 sets is all that's needed.

SUPERSET THESE TWO EXERCISES

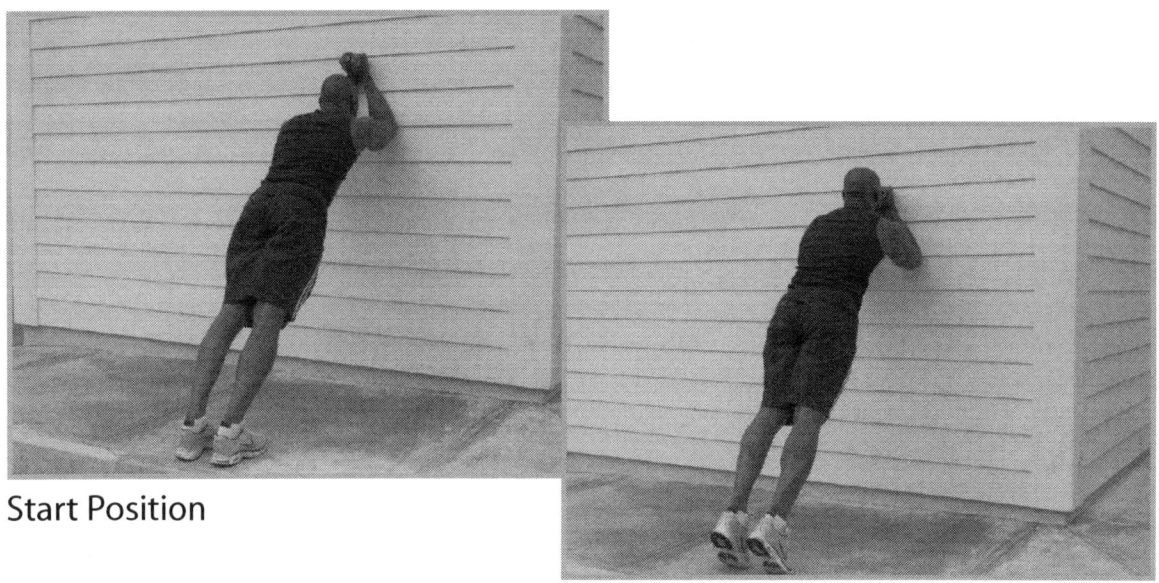

Start Position

Finished Position

Superset Workout Continued.......

Standing Calve Raises

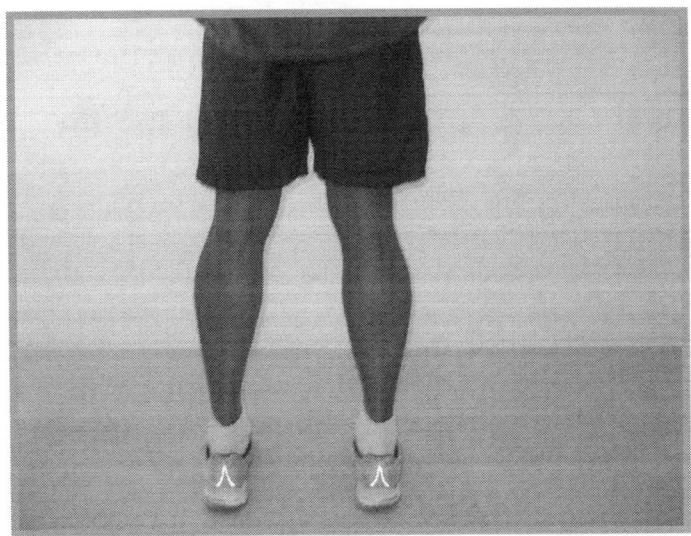

Start Position

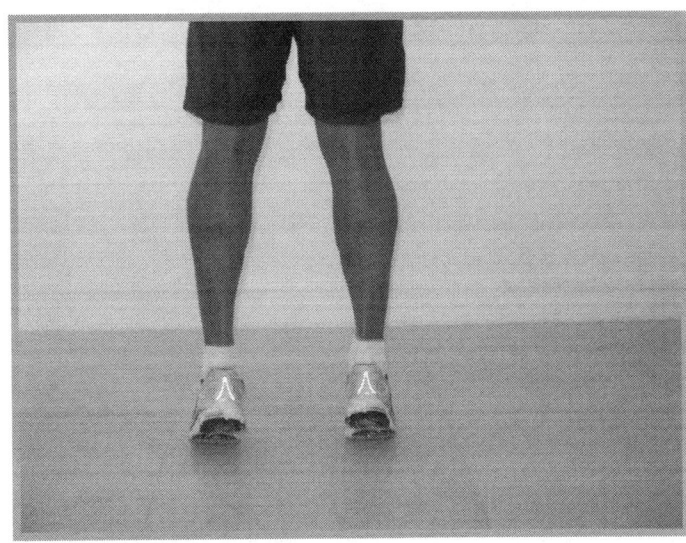

Finished Position

This combination increases blood blocking occlusion to increase capillary development in the calve wall structure.
Perform 20 reps each at 3 sets

ABS

Superset Routine One

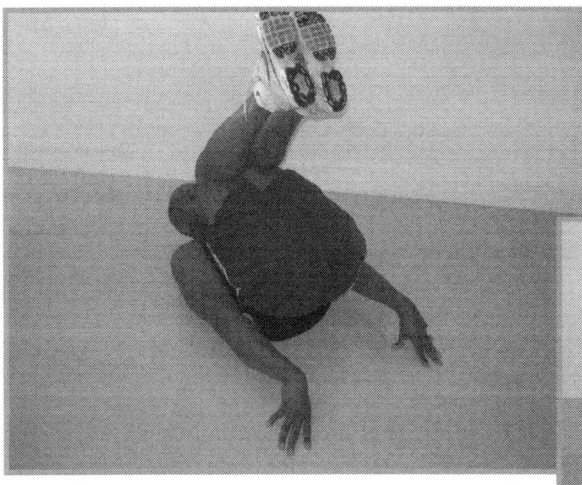

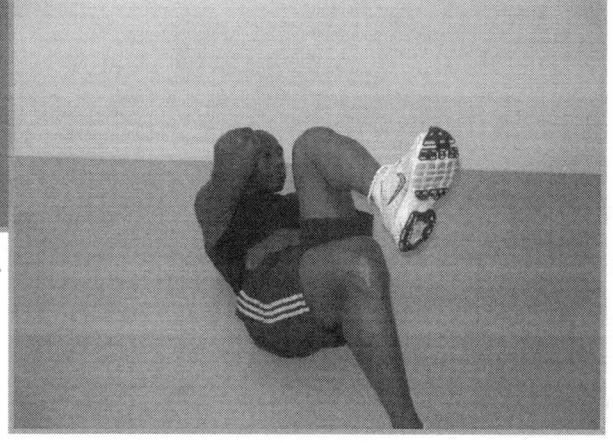

Perform 15-20 reps each 4 rounds. Rest 5 seconds after the first two exercises are completed.

Superset Routine Two

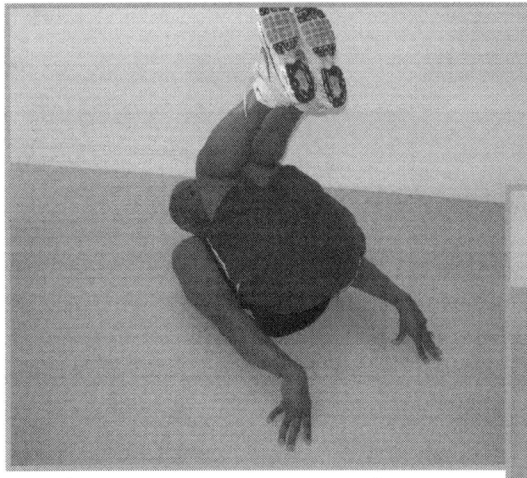

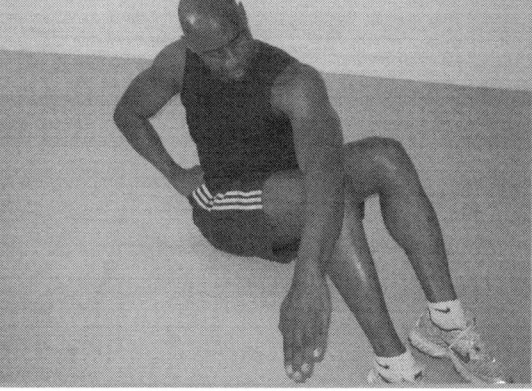

Perform 15-20 reps each 4 rounds. Rest 5 seconds after first two exercises are completed.

Chapter 7

EVERY OTHER DAY ROUTINE PLUS ARM SPECIALIZATION
FIBER-OVERLOAD TRAINING METHOD Tuesday Thursday and Saturday
Workout Perform 3 weeks

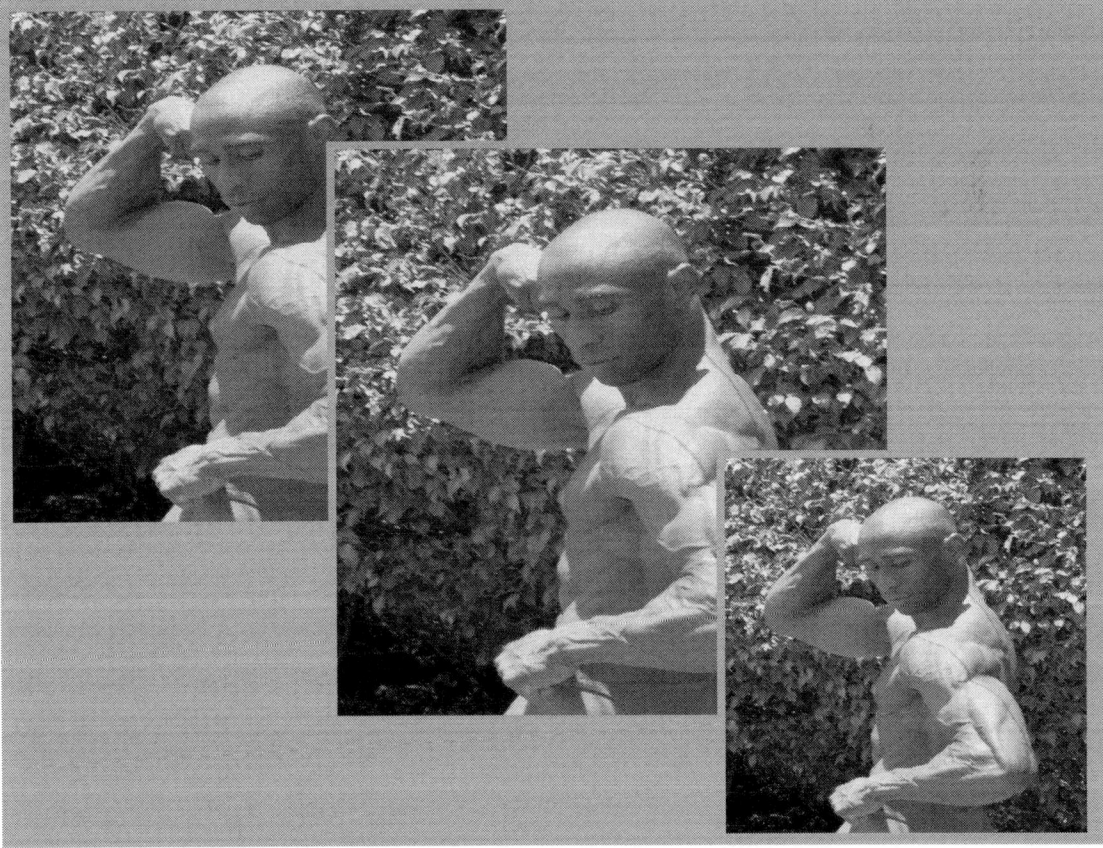

CHAPTER 7

EVERY OTHER DAY ROUTINE PLUS ARM SPECIALIZATION
FIBER OVERLOAD TRAINING METHOD
Tuesday Thursday and Saturday Workout Perform 3 weeks

Nothing commands more respect than an awesome pair of rock hard chiseled arms that hang off the shoulders. So let's get to it....

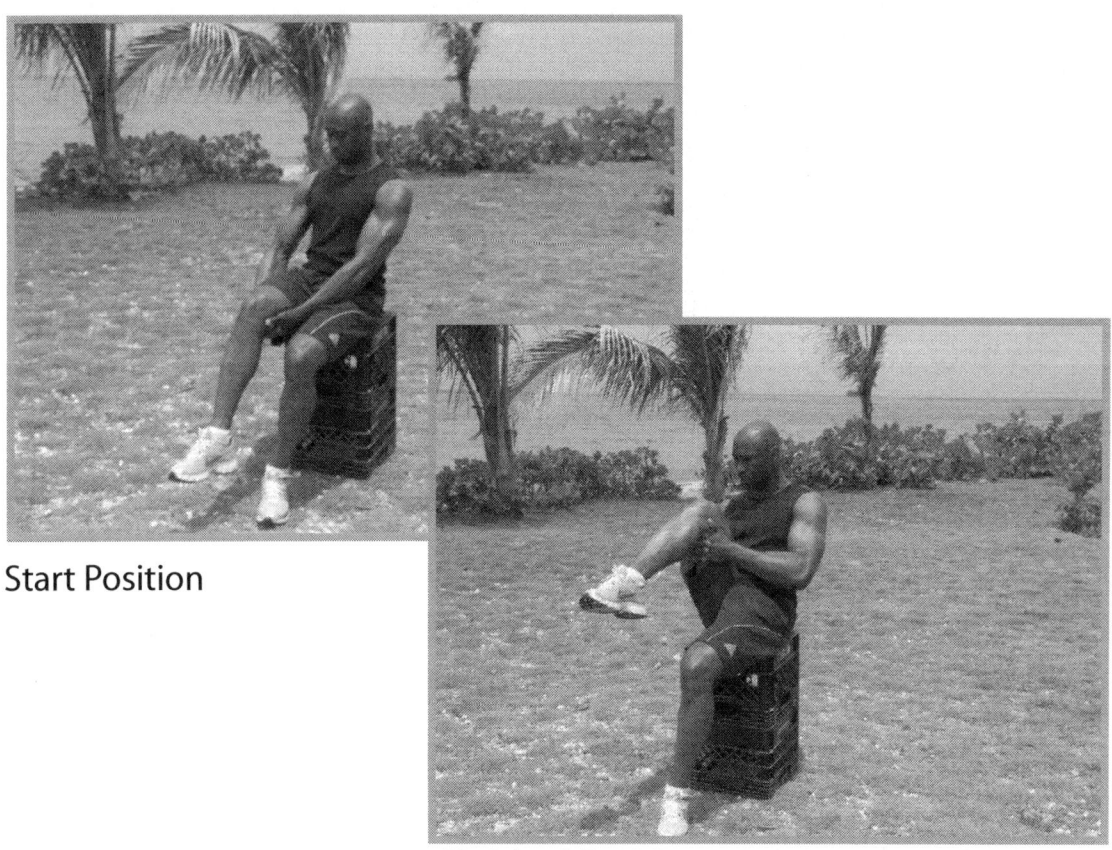

Start Position

Finished Position

This is where muscle-team-work comes in to make the bicep contract at it's maximum! In the seated position interlock the fingers behind the knee and using the bicep strength pull the leg towards the chest while resisting with that leg. Great for the biceps, forearms, and upper back. Do not push the leg down. Just relax and try it again.
It's best performed at 3 sets of 15 reps.

Reverse Curls

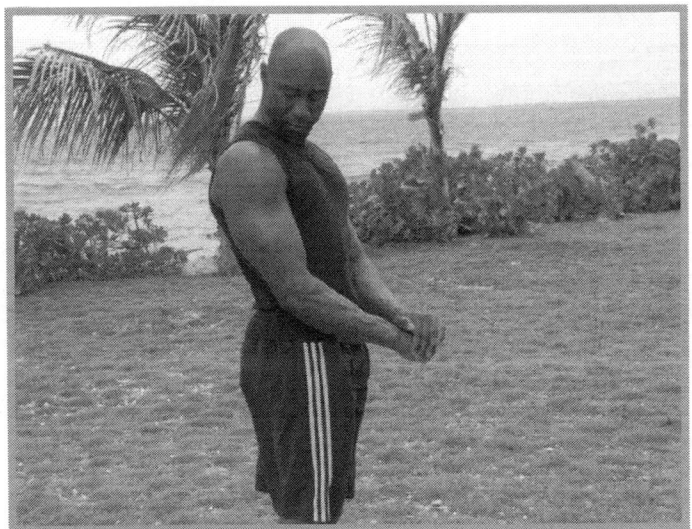

Start Position

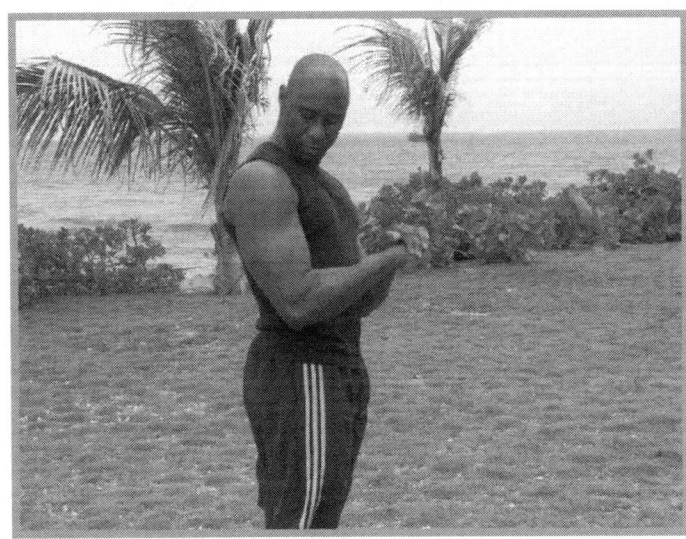

Finished Position

Reverse curls are done in the same manner resisting in both ranges to the mid-point of the exercise stroke. Perform 3 sets 12-15 reps.

Overhead Bicep Curls

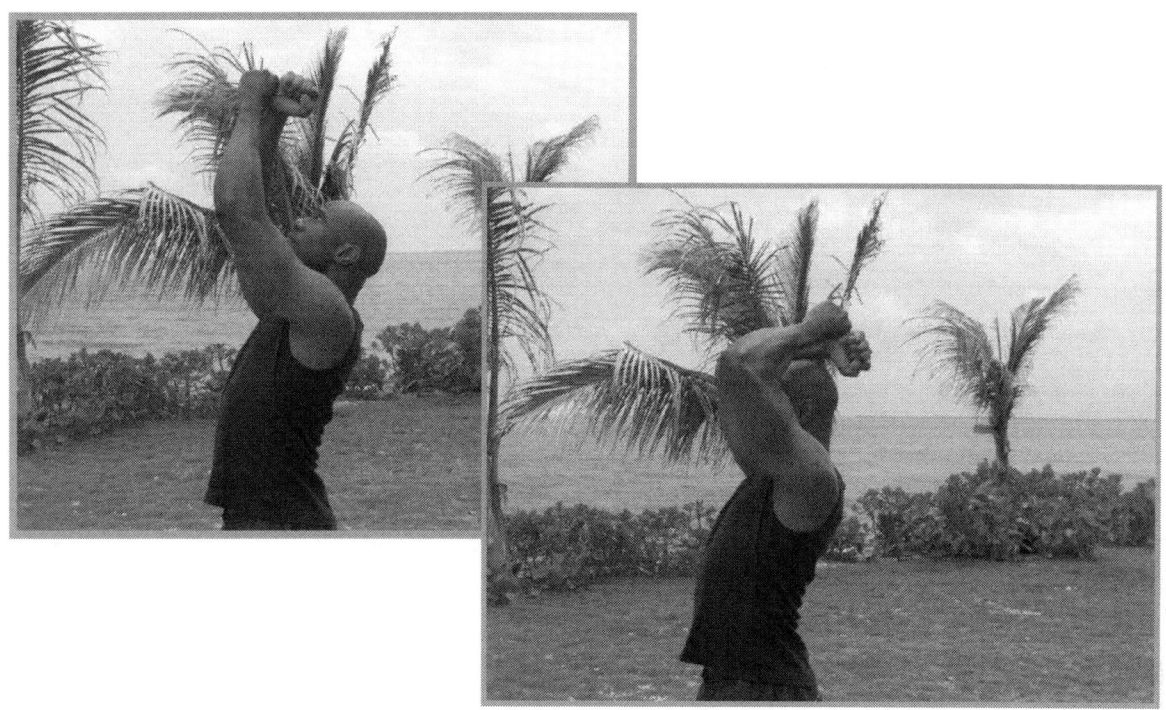

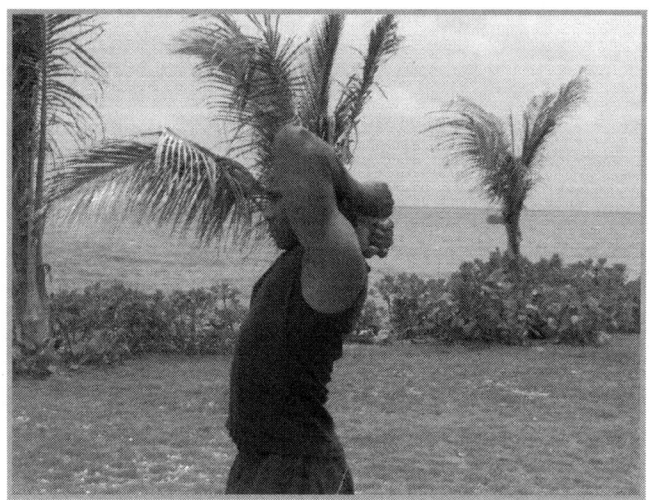

Now this is a very powerful bicep developer! We are talking high peak biceps here. Use a moderate tension and resist on the down stroke only. Perform the full range, relax and start again same arm. 3 sets 15 reps.

Triceps

Tricep Pressdown

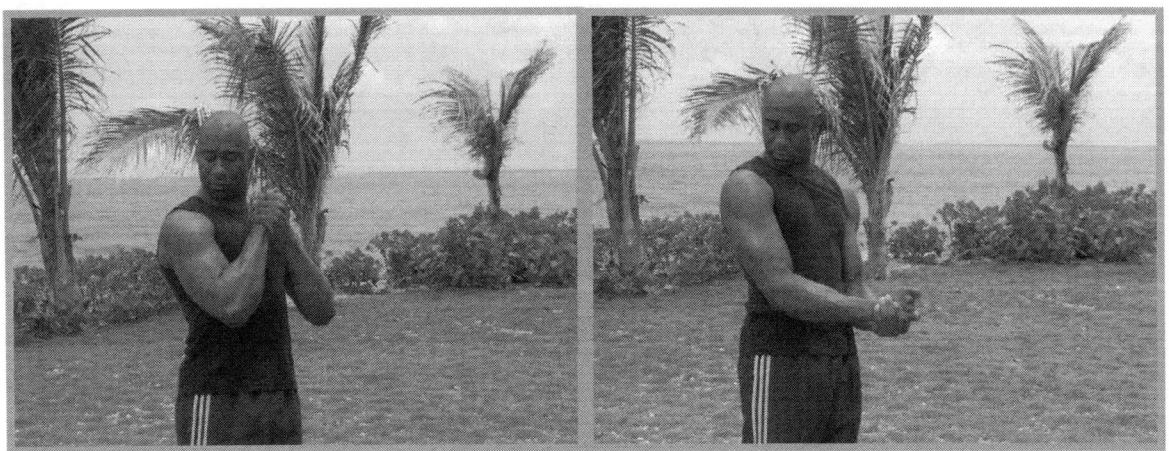

Start Position Finished Position

Now here's the real deal. Time to make the long head of the triceps flare out! The strongest signal again Mid-Point. Perform 3 sets of 15-18 reps resisting on the down movement Only.

Forward Lateral Press

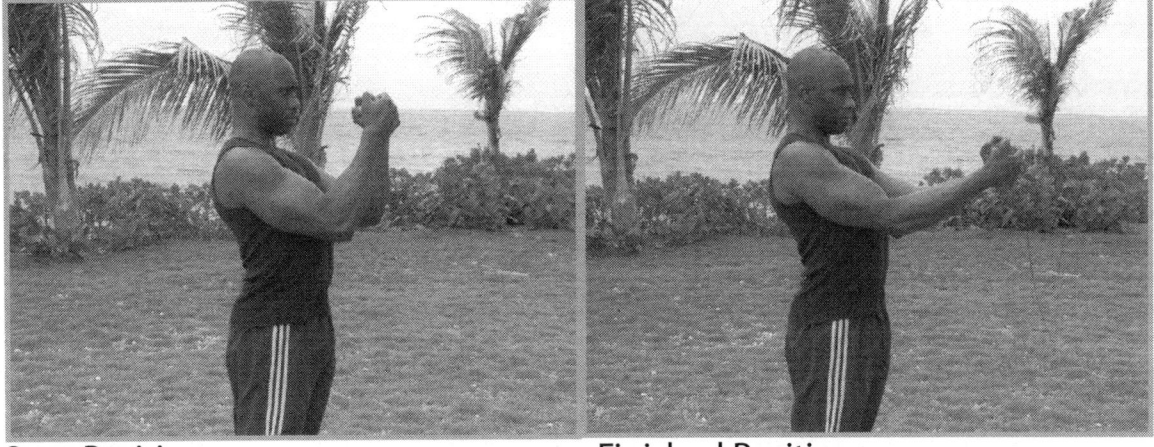

Start Position Finished Position

Start the position at the middle of the exercise stroke and press the arm forward maintaining tension by keeping the elbow bent. Then pull the arm back. In other words Resist in both directions. Perform 3 sets of 15-18 reps

Over Head Press

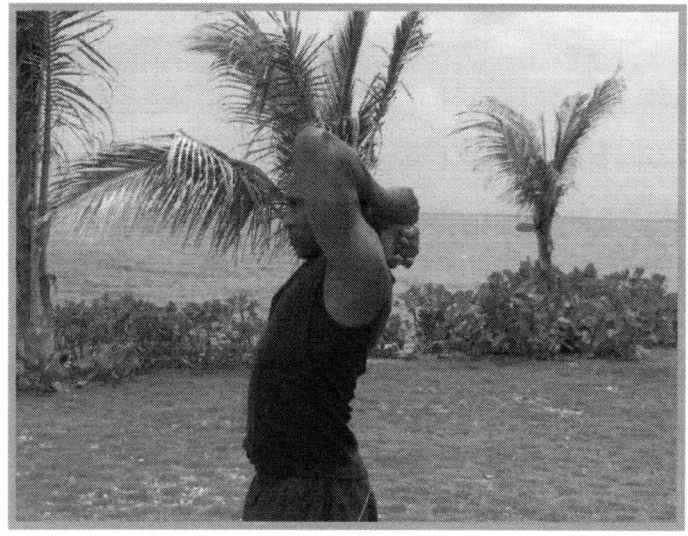

Start Position

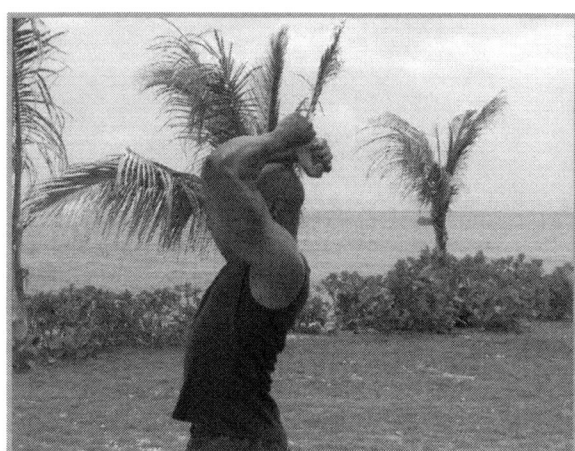

Mid-Point

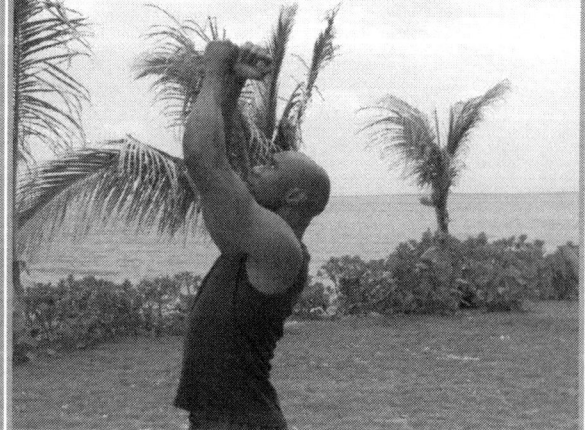

Finished Position

Full reps are done with this one. Remember don't use too much force, for this exercise place the tendons of the elbows in a very sensitive Position. Resist both ways for desired reps then switch. 3 sets of 15 reps is all you need.

Monday Wednesday Friday

This is the other section of this routine

Across-The-Body Pulls

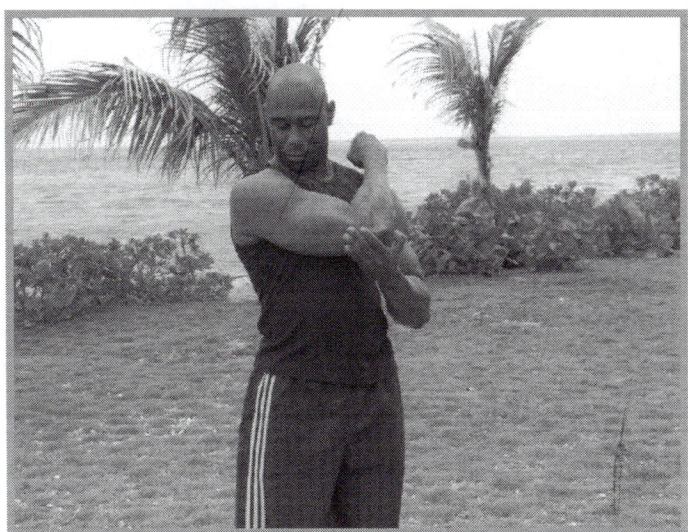

Start Position

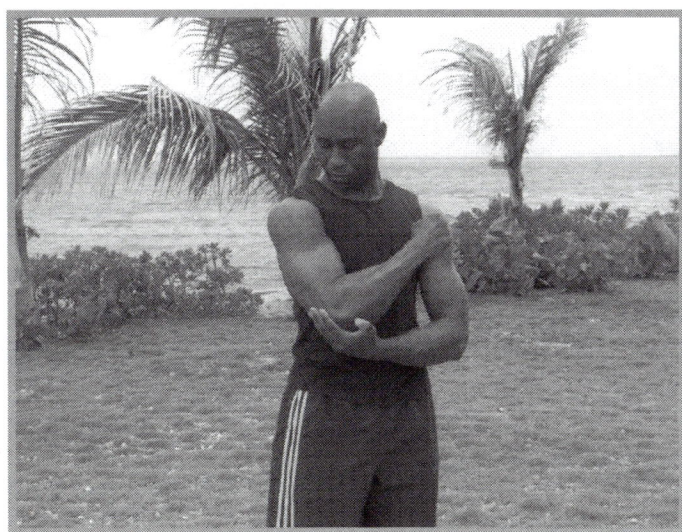

Finished Position

Perform 3 sets of 15 reps of this exercise. Rest time can be 5 seconds when both shoulders are done. Resist in one direction Only.

Upper Back

Stiff-Arm-Pulldowns

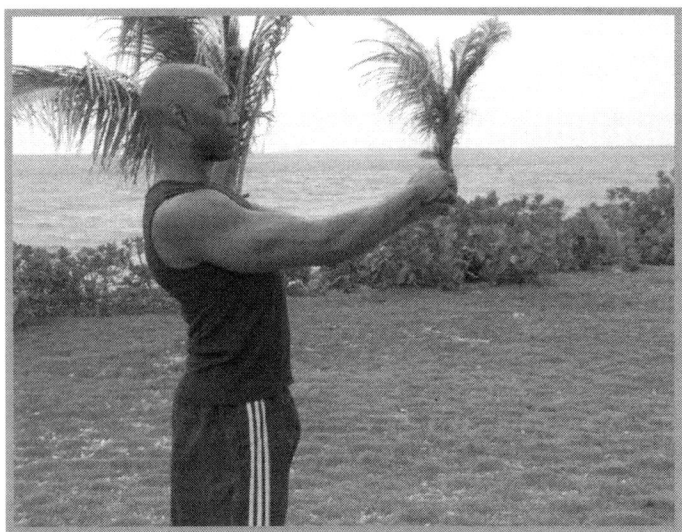

Start Position

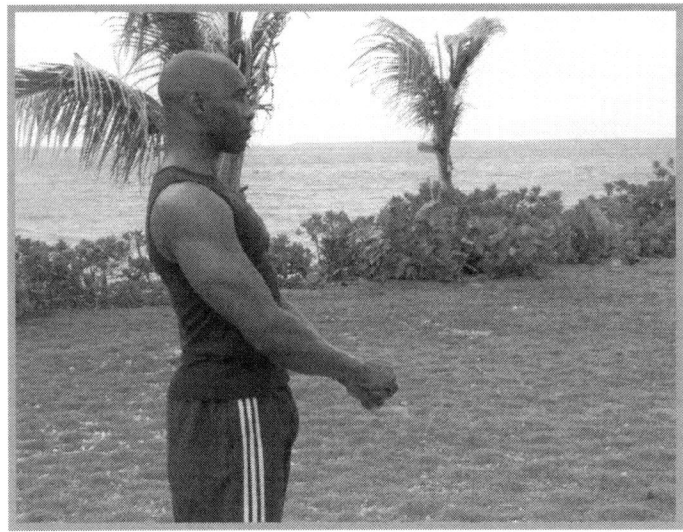

Finished Position

Resist in both directions. 15 reps 3 sets each side.

Chest

Three Chair Pushups

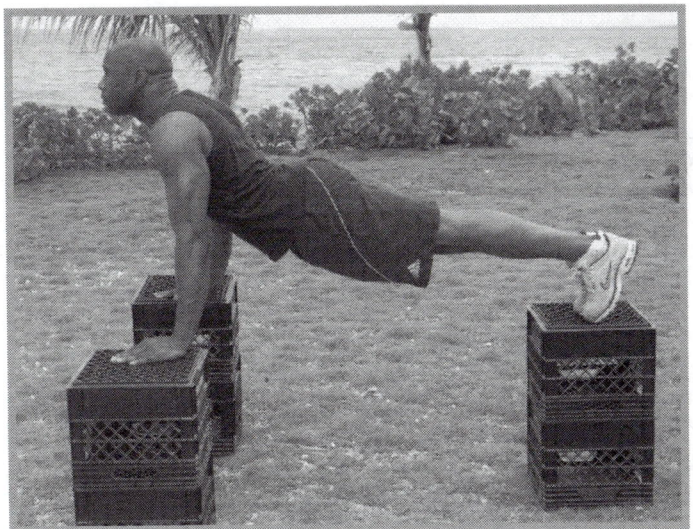

Start Position

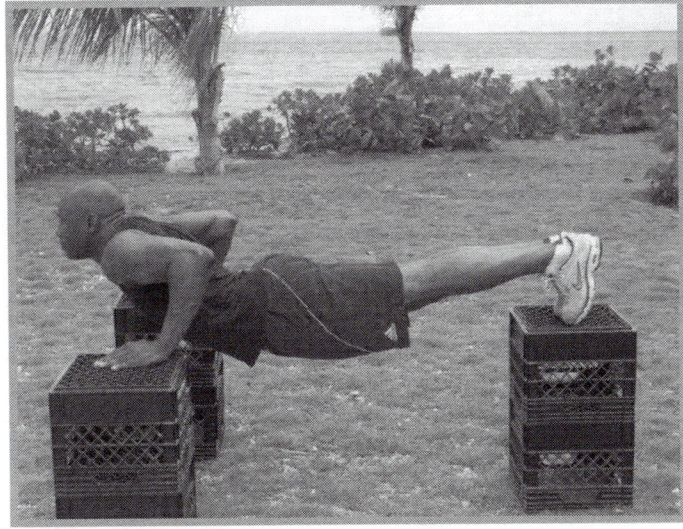

Finished Position

Three Chair Pushups are quite similar to the decline pushups. Same instruction pause for a few seconds at the bottom to increase the pre-stretch but only stop to the point of stretch. Don't over stretch. Then press upwards again maintaining a slight bend to the elbows to maintain tension on the muscle at hand. Perform 3 sets of 15 reps

Decline Pushups

Decline Pushups

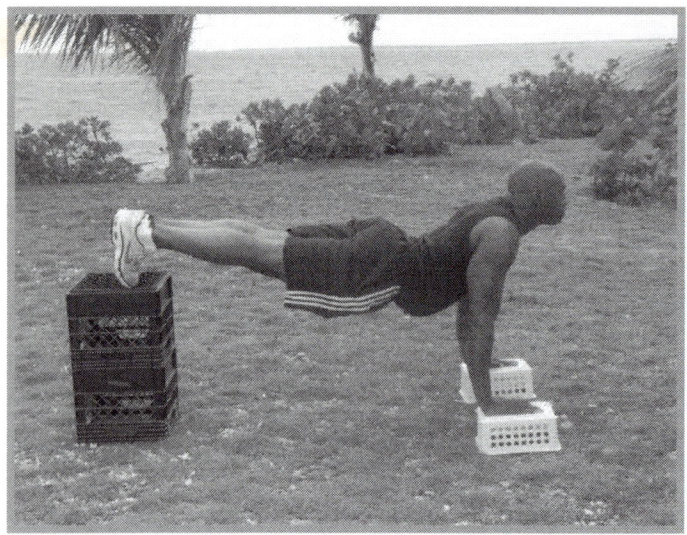

Start Position

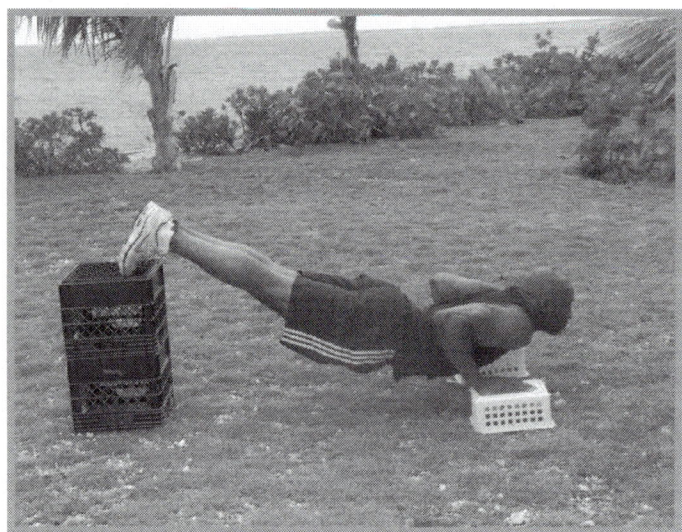

Finished Position

Pause at the bottom position for a few seconds then press back up to the start position. Perform 15 reps at 3-4 sets

Liederman Press

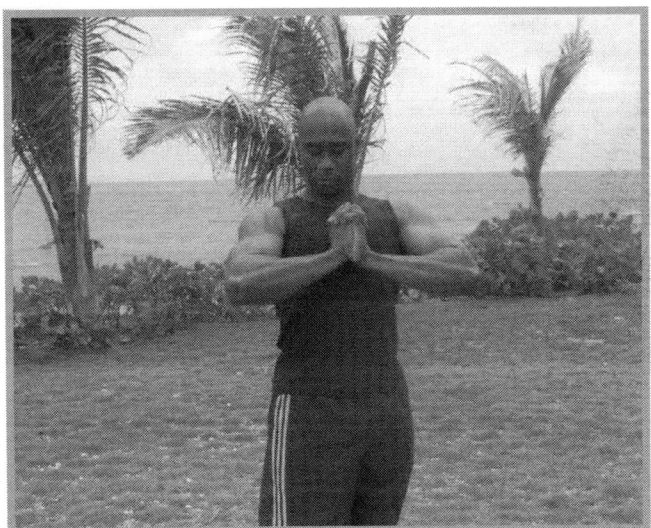

Start Position

Perform 15 reps of 3-4 sets each. Pausing at the end of each rep at the shoulder for 2-3 seconds before reversing the movement.

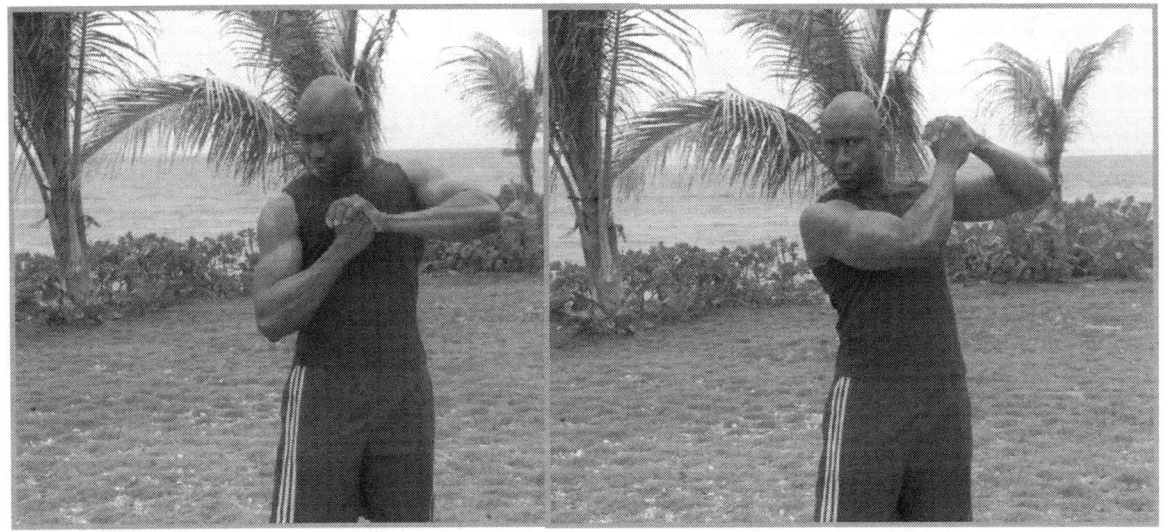

Start Position   Finished Position

A new one for you guys resist in one position only. Perform 3 sets of 12-15 reps. This is a fine exercise for the upper chest, shoulders and triceps.

Upper Chest Press

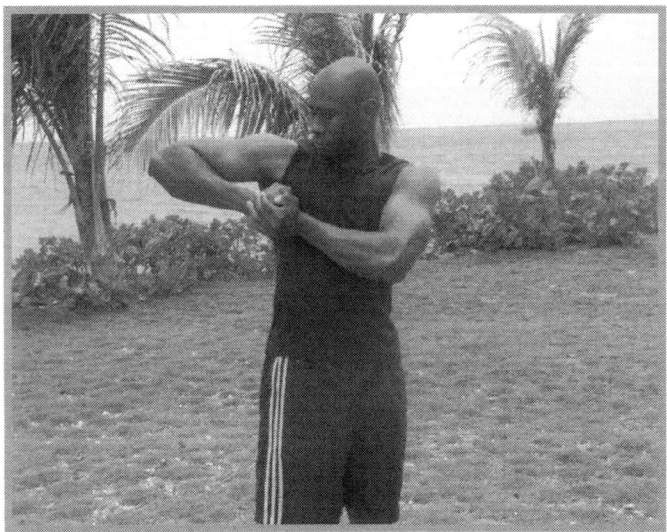

Start Position

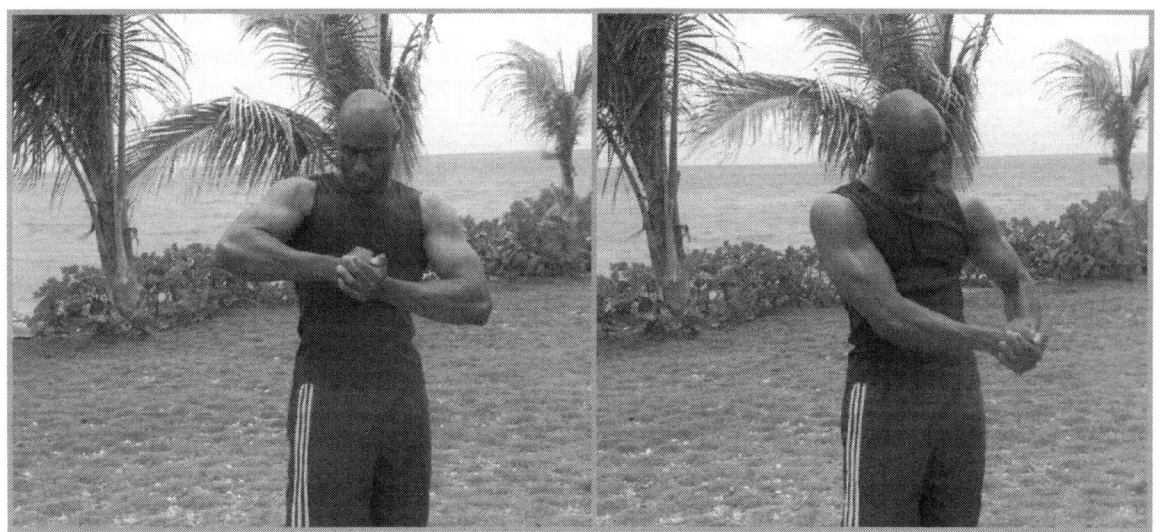

Mid-Point   Finished Position

Perform this exercise resisting in both directions but (Focus) on the downward movement! Perform as shown in pictures 15 reps with the right arm then repeat another 15 with the left. 3 sets each arm. Complete both sides and rest 5 seconds and continue.

Shoulders

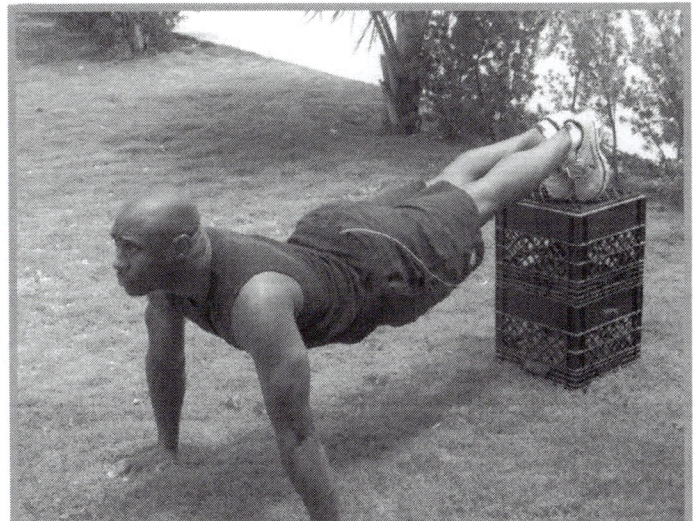

Start Position

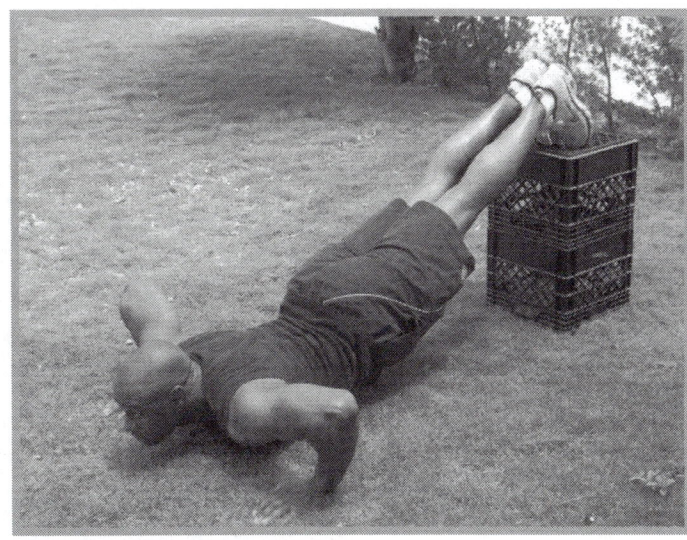

Finished Position

Perform exercise as shown pausing at the bottom position for 2-3 seconds to increase the pre-stretch and HGH production. Then reverse the exercise by pressing back upwards maintaining a slight bend to the elbow. 15 reps at 3-4 sets are all that you need for this movement.

Neck

Rear Neck press

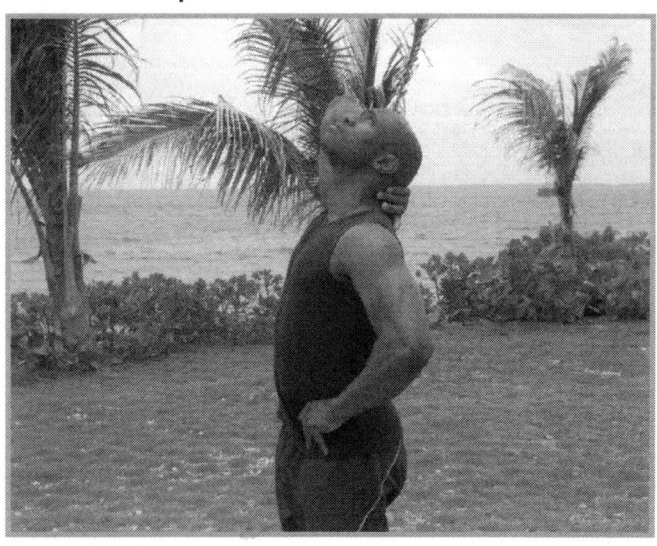

Side to Side Neck Press   Front Neck Press

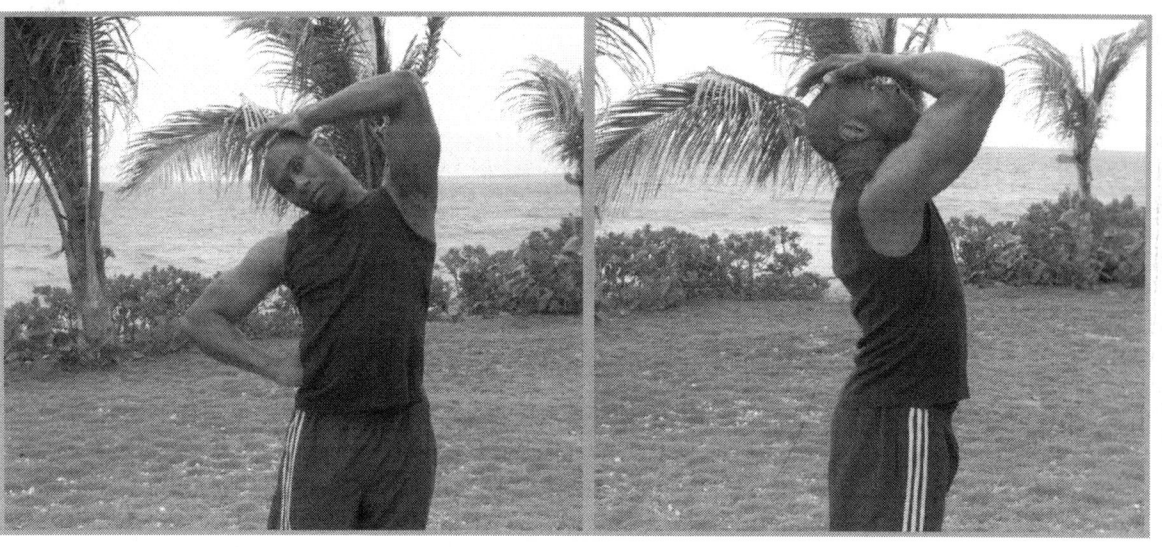

You know the drills here. Resist in one direction 20 reps 3 sets each movement.

Hamstrings/Thighs

Resisted Thigh and Hamstring Combo

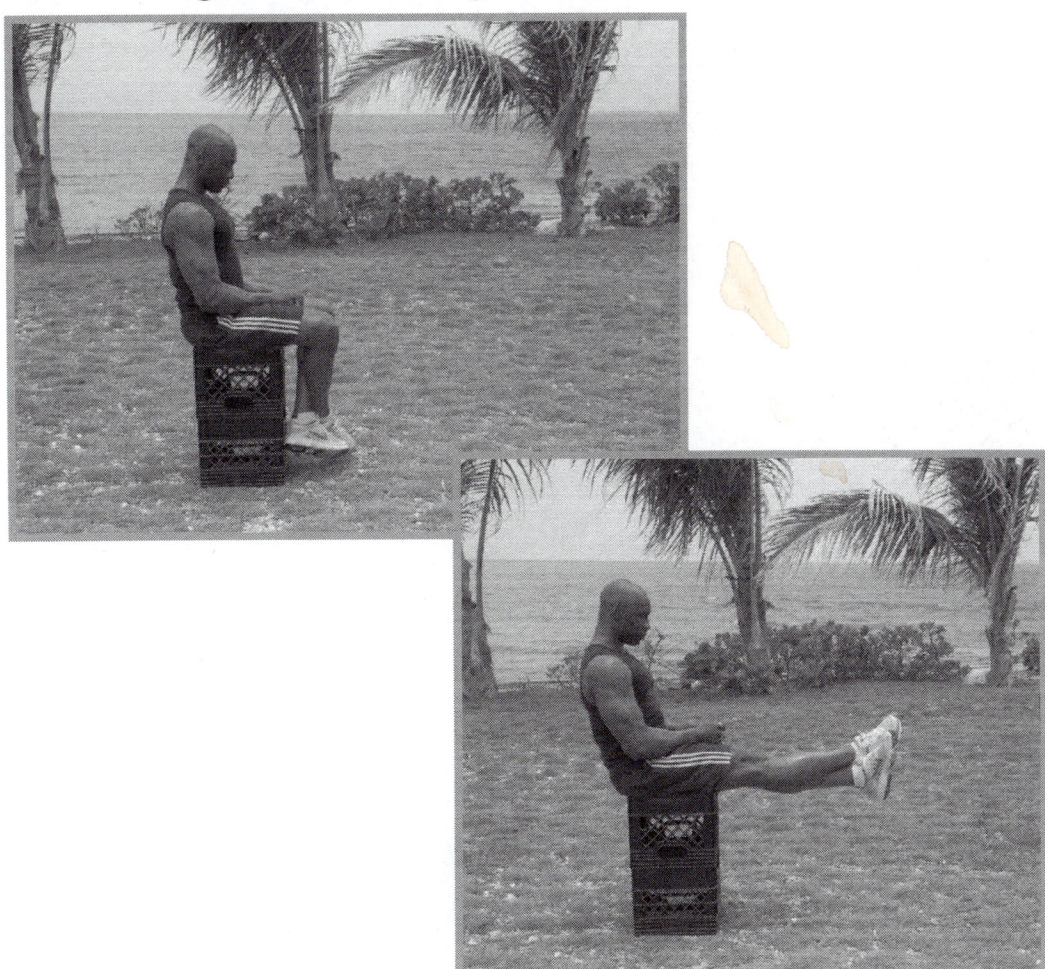

This time resist in both directions both thighs and hamstring combo. Perform desired reps then switch legs. 15 reps at 3 sets each leg.

Thighs (Basic)

Regular Squats

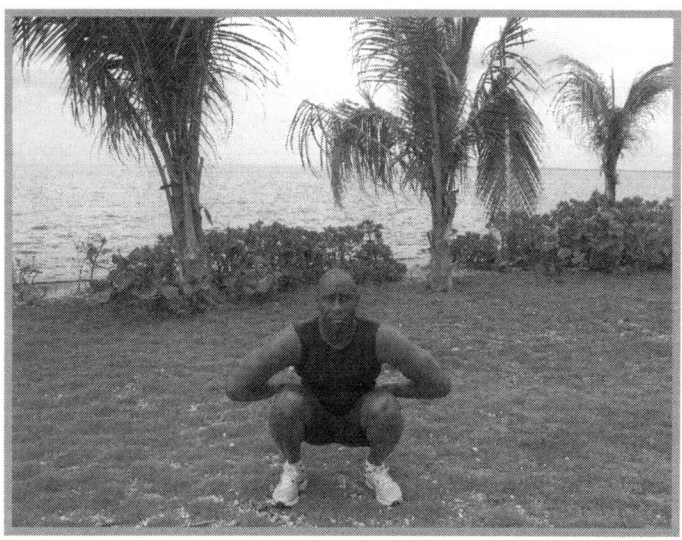

Crossed Legged Squats

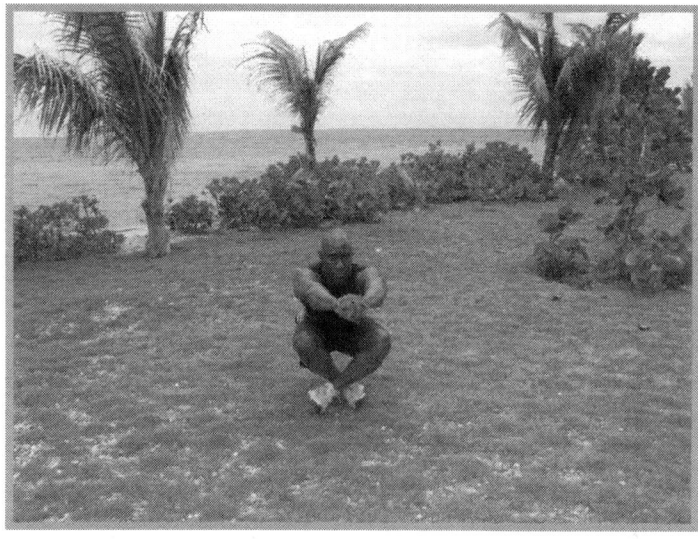

All Squating movements are to be done at 20 reps 3 sets each. Rest between sets 5-10 seconds. Maintain a slight bend at the knees in standing position.

Forearms

Forearm Press

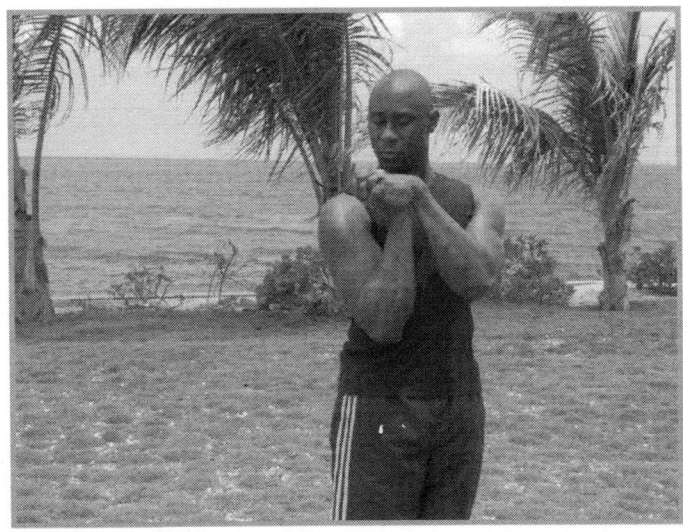

Palm Up Wrist Curls

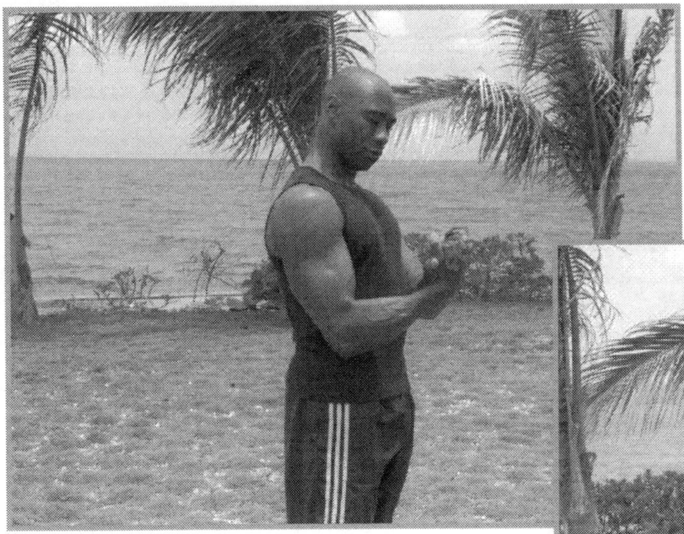

Palm Down Wrist Curls

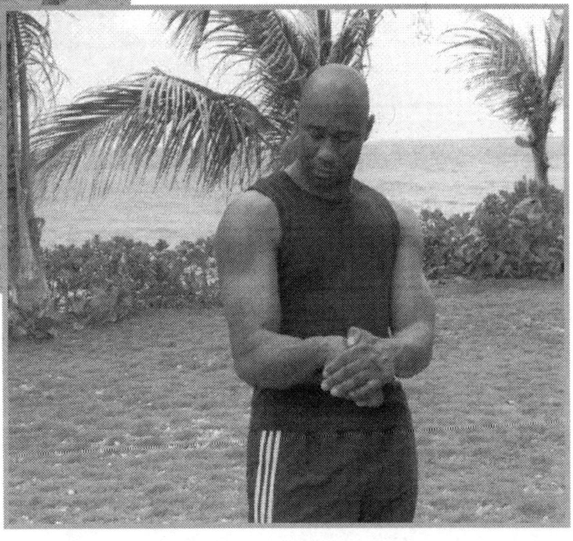

Perform the forearm exercises resisting back and forth for desired reps. 20 reps each exercise 3 sets each. Rest time between sets (None)

Standing Calve Raises

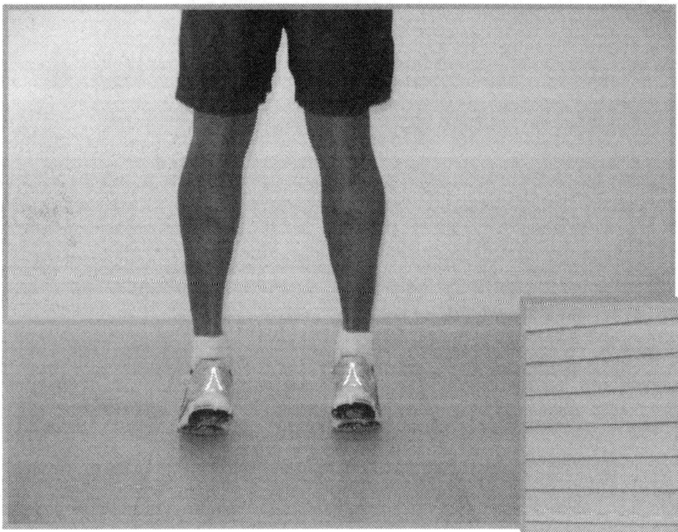

Slanted Calve Raises

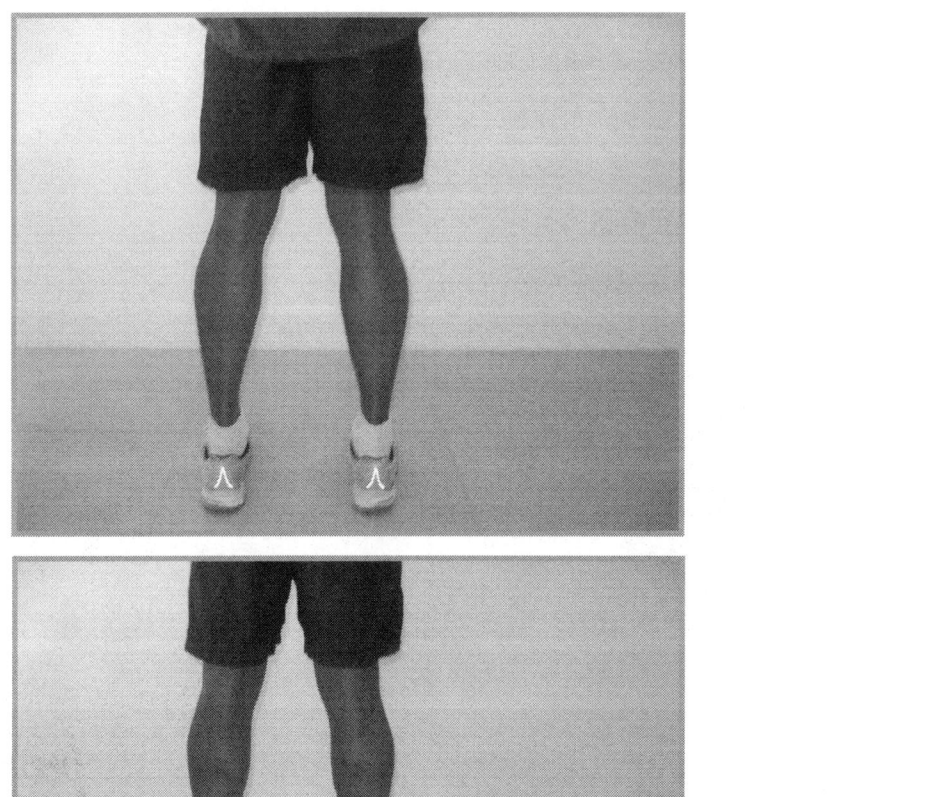

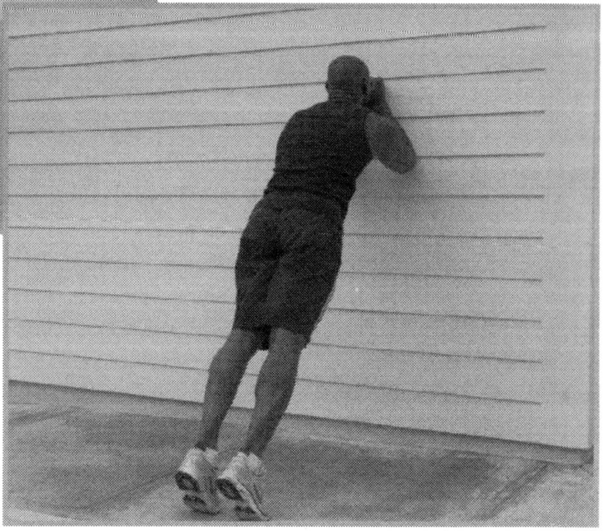

Same Drills as before 20 reps, 3 sets each. No Rest between exercises

Specialization Routine Two

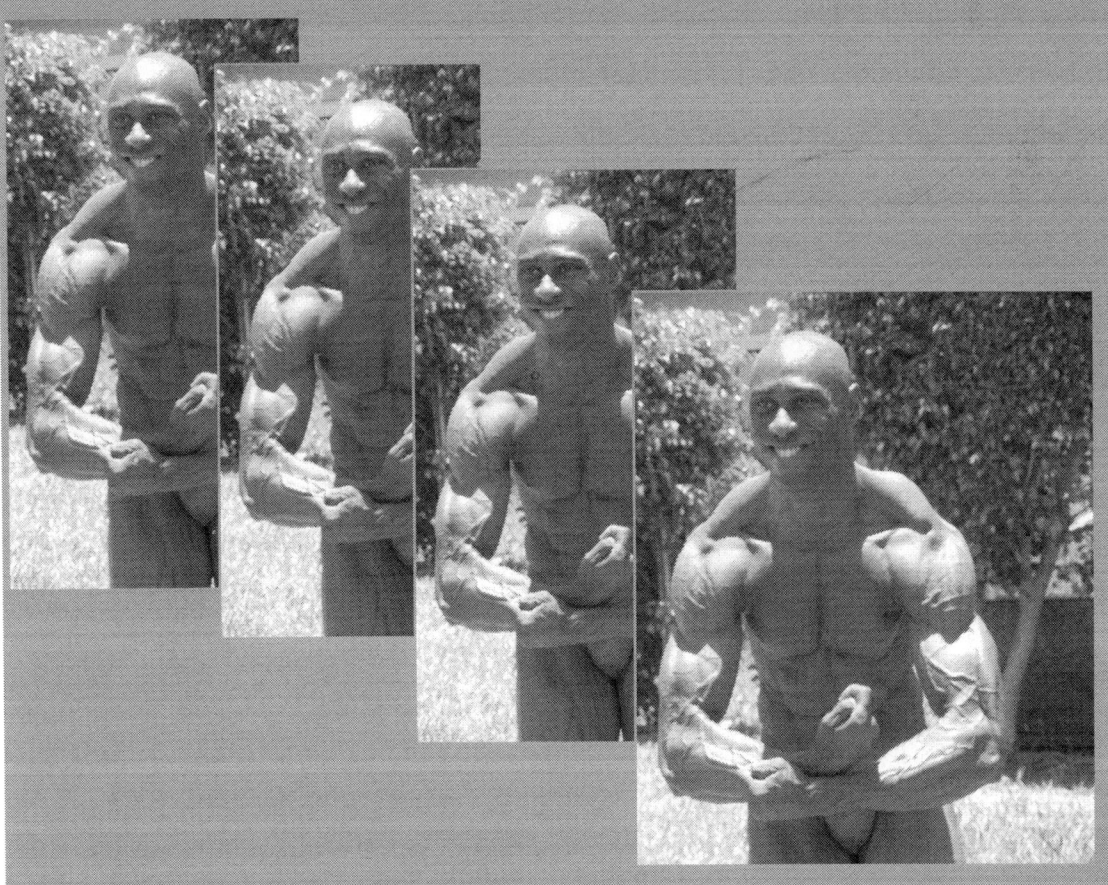

Specialization Routine Two

After 3 weeks of the specialized arm routine try this arm routine with any of the phases for another 3-4 weeks

We start off with this exercise again. The Thigh Rows to increase force on the biceps with muscle-team-work. Perform 2 sets of 12 reps per side. As this warms up the targeted muscle (biceps)

Thigh Rows

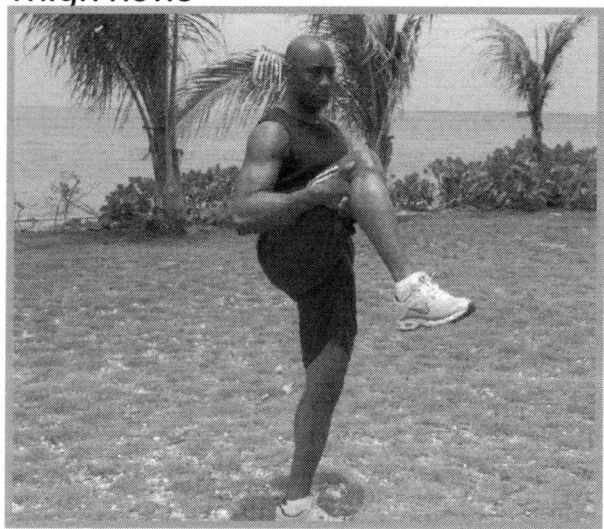

When this is done, perform the three bicep exercises listed on the other page. Working the three exercises first on the right arm for desired reps then switching to the other arm for another three exercises.
Pause and repeat the sequence again.

Performing 12-15 reps each exercise at 3 sets each before switching arms. Resist in both directions.

Biceps

Palm-Up Curl

Reverse Curls

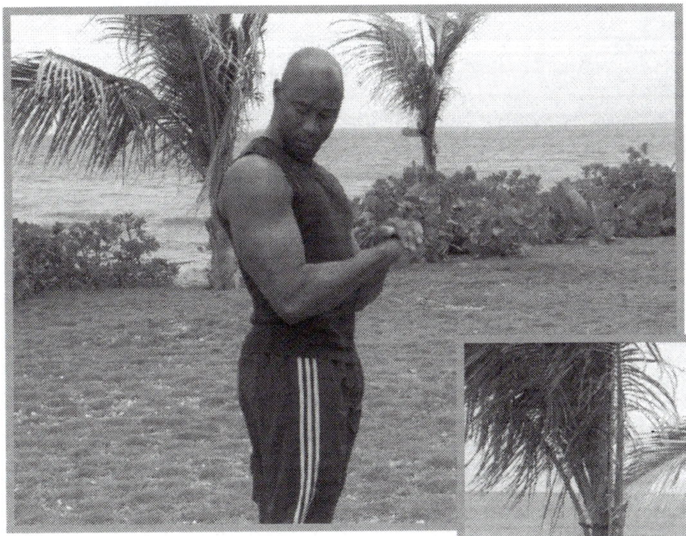

Hammer Curls

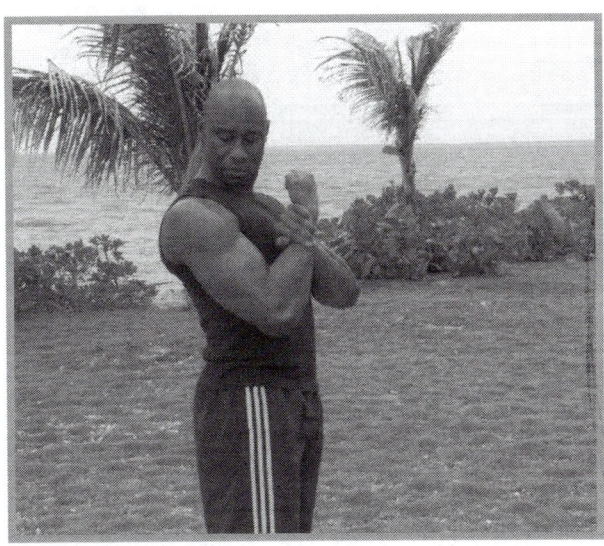

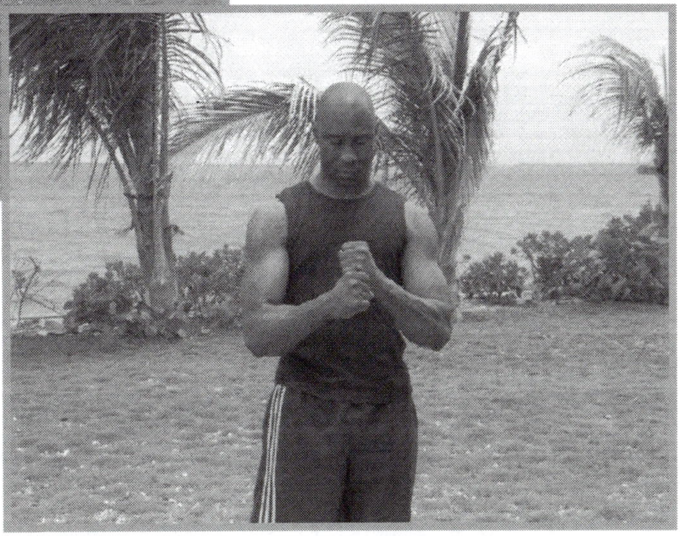

After your combo is completed. It's concentration curls. This stimulates the target muscle in the peak contraction and forces the muscle to contract with greater force. Perform 20 reps per side at 2 sets each arm. Resisting in both directions.

Concentration Curls

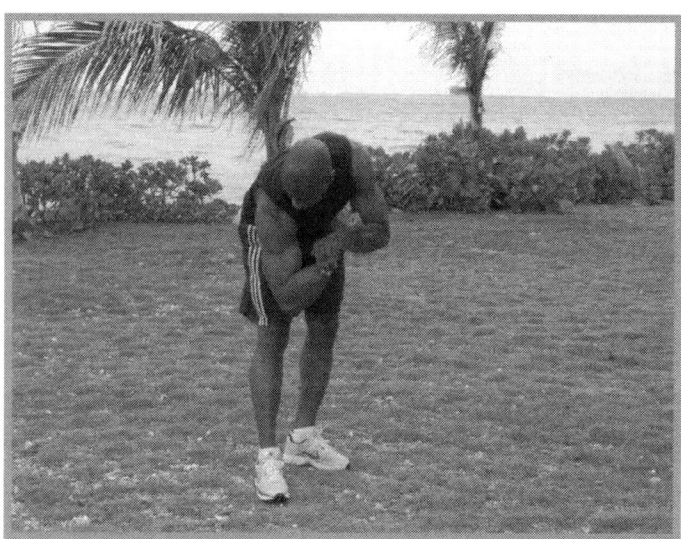

Forearms

Palm Up Wrist Curl

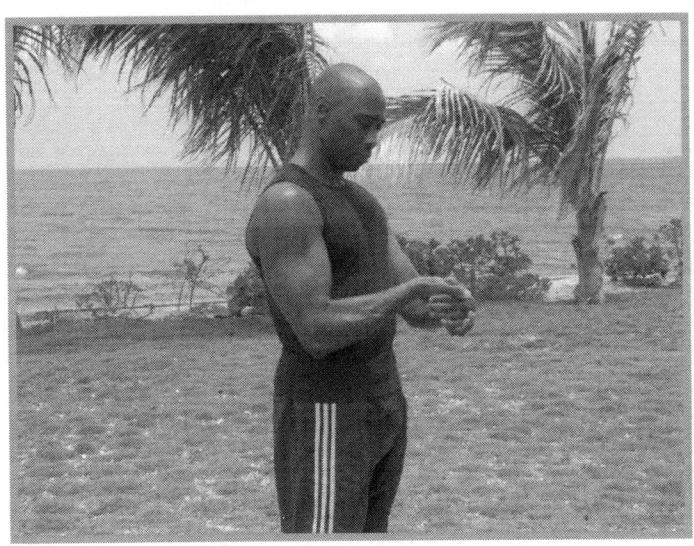

Palm Down Wrist Curls

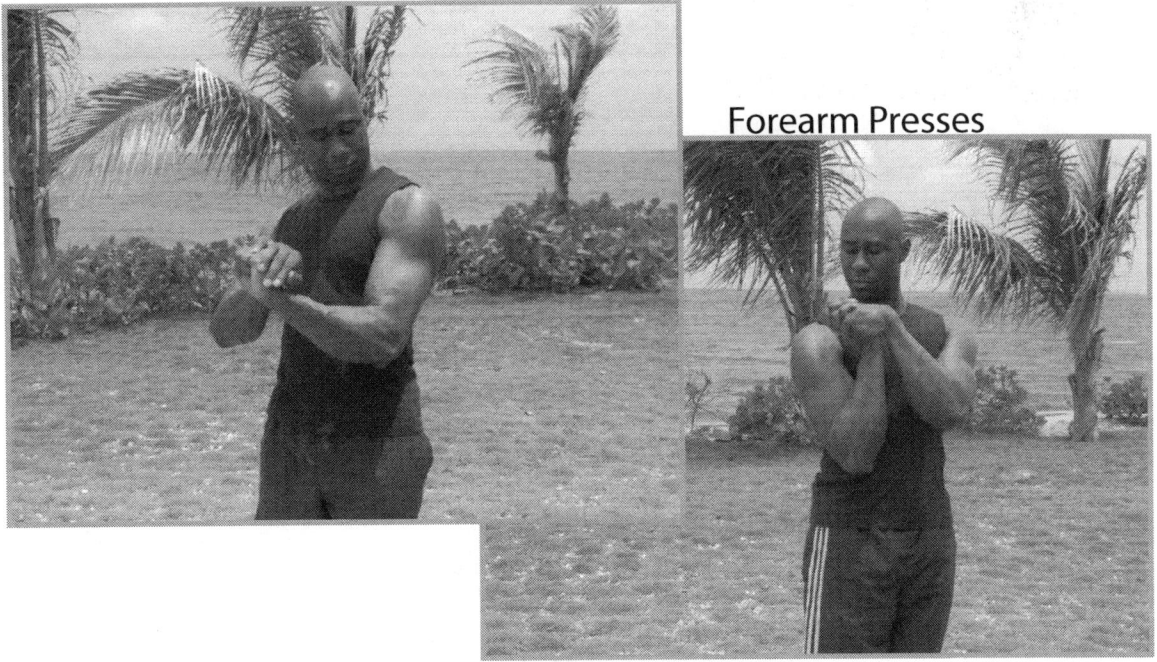

Forearm Presses

Forearm exercises are done in the very same manner. Three exercises back to back then switch hands. 20 reps at 3 sets is enough.

Triceps

Forward Lateral Press

Tricep Pressdown

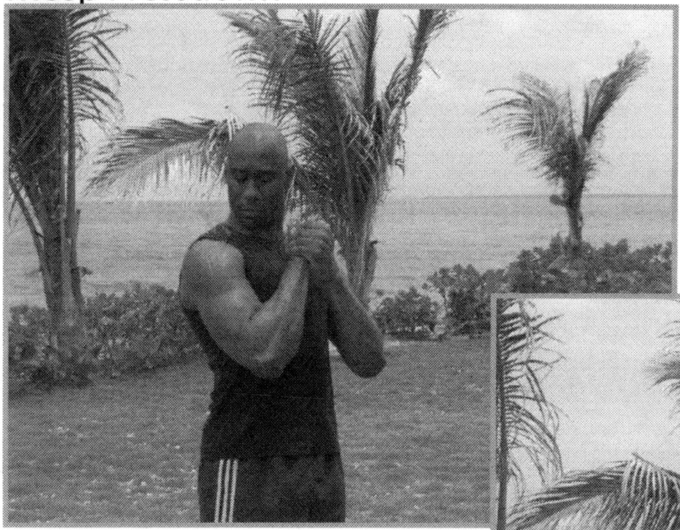

Overhead Tricep Press

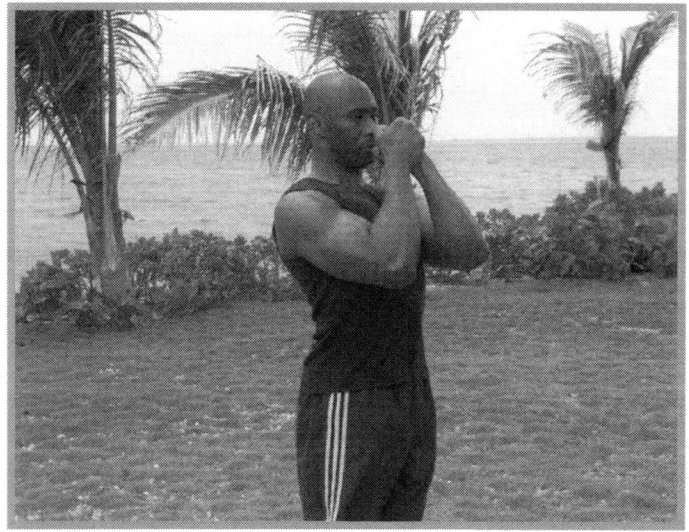

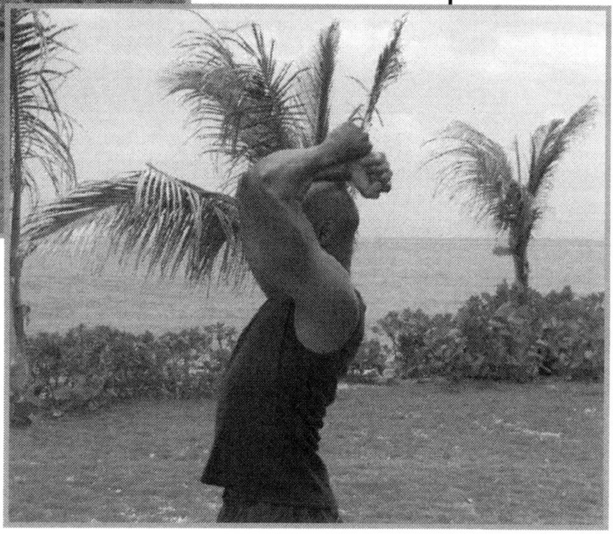

Again for the triceps perform three exercises immediately after each other for desired reps, then switch arms and repeat sequence. Perform 12-15 reps each exercise at 3 sets each.

Triceps

Decline Extensions

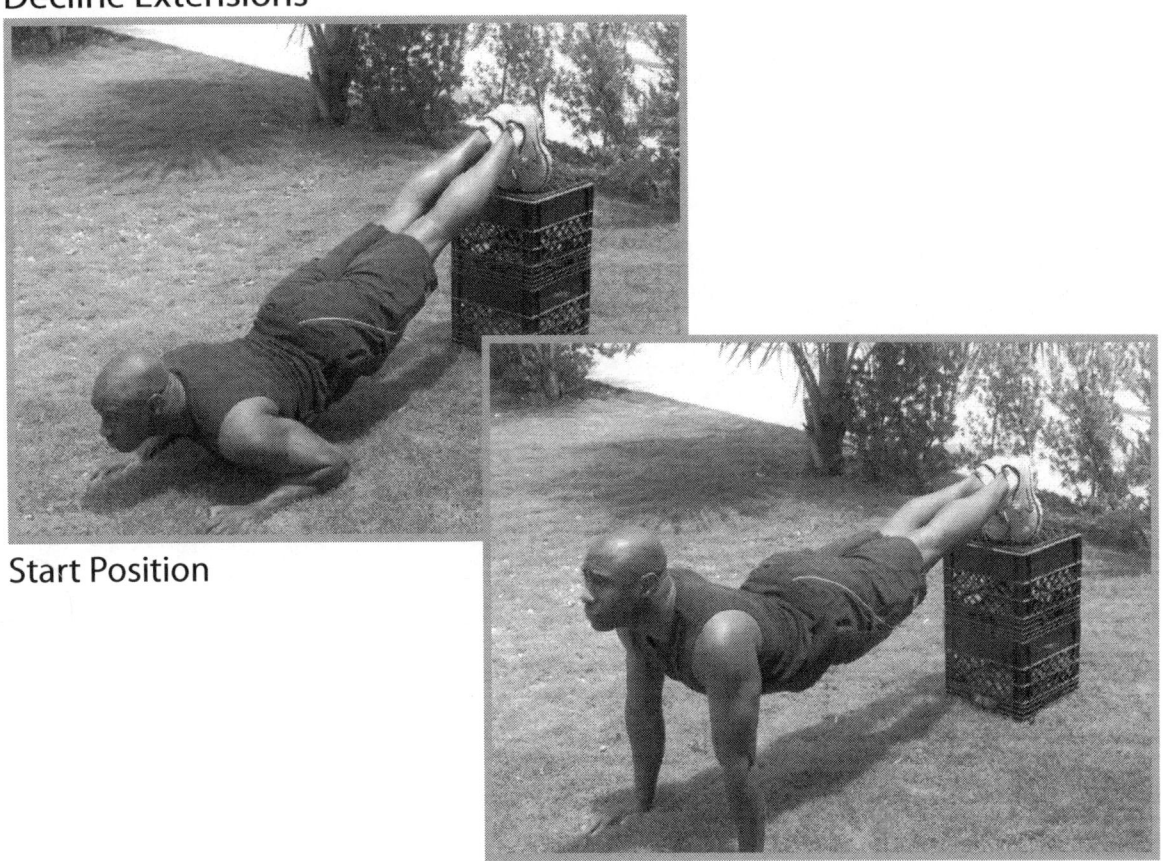

Start Position

Finished Position

After the tricep combo, it's decline extensions. Perform 7-12 reps at 3 sets. Maintaining a slight bend at the elbow in the finished position. Excellent! There you've got it. This is an Introductory mini course to The Beyond Self Resistance Bodybuilding Manual If you enjoyed this book it was only a teaser to an in-dept version of Beyond Self Resistance. Contact Me On Your Progress at

skippymarl@cwky.blackberry.net

Anytime. Keep at it and Expect Success.

Marlon Birch

Made in the USA
Lexington, KY
16 September 2015